Fibromyalgia

Fibromyalgia

A NATURAL APPROACH

Christine Craggs-Hinton

Ulysses Press — Berkeley, CA

2004

Published by: Ulysses Press
P.O. Box 3440
Berkeley, CA 94703
www.ulyssespress.com

Library of Congress Catalog Card Number: 2003104409
ISBN: 1-56975-369-5

First published in the United Kingdom in 2001 as *Living with Fibromyalgia* and *The Fibromyalgia Healing Diet* by Sheldon Press

Printed in Canada by Transcontinental Printing

10 9 8 7 6 5 4 3 2 1

Editor: Richard Harris
Cover Design: Sarah Levin
Cover Photo: copyright Photos.com
Editorial and production staff: Kate Allen, Laura Brancella, Lily Chou, Claire Chun, Leslie Henriques, Lisa Kester, Lynette Ubois
Indexer: Sayre Van Young

Distributed in the United States by Publishers Group West and in Canada by Raincoast Books

All names and identifying characteristics of real persons have been changed in the text to protect their confidentiality.

NOTE FROM THE PUBLISHER
This book has been written and published strictly for informational purposes, and in no way should it be used as a substitute for consultation with your medical doctor or health care professional. All facts in this book came from medical files, clinical journals, scientific publications, personal interviews, published trade books, self-published materials by experts, magazine articles, and the personal-practice experiences of the authorities quoted or sources cited. You should not consider educational material herein to be the practice of medicine or to replace consultation with a physician or other medical practitioner. The author and publisher are providing you with information in this work so that you can have the knowledge and can choose, at your own risk, to act on that knowledge. The author and publisher also urge all readers to be aware of their health status and to consult health professionals before beginning any health program, including changes in dietary habits.

Contents

Dedication

This book is dedicated to my husband, David, and to my late father, Ernest Chamberlain.

Without the love, support and encouragement of David I would not be the "together" person I am today, neither would I have had the confidence to research and write a book such as this.

Without my father's enduring sense of fun and determination to make the most of his lot—even in the worst days of his own illness—I would not have had the example that has helped me cope with my fibromyalgia.

I would like to mention my three boys, too—Mark, James and Matthew Earley. Absolute horrors when they were younger (only joking) they are now wonderful, caring young men I am incredibly proud to call my own. Thank you, boys, for being so good to your old mum!

Acknowledgments

I would like to say special thanks to:

Dr. R. N. Ashworth, my former GP;

Mavis Bannan, my very close friend, who recently died after a long struggle with cancer, for, despite her illness, she generously offered her help and support in all my ventures and throughout the worst days of my own illness—I will never forget her enormous kindness and bravery;

Glenn Chamberlain, my brother, who, despite his handicaps, has a heart of gold and would pull the moon from the sky for his big sister;

Mabel Chamberlain, my mother, for helping to edit my work and being a good friend;

Dr. Mary Cuthbert, my GP, for her compassion and understanding of my condition;

David Fairfax, a homeopathic practitioner, whose remedies have helped to keep me going;

Margaret Gray, Chairperson of the Fibromyalgia Support and Carers' Group (West Yorkshire), for her selfless devotion to fibromyalgics in this area and her hard work on behalf of our group;

Dr. J. Raphael, Consultant specializing in pain management and member of the Fibromyalgia Association UK Board of Trustees, who kindly verified my medical data;

Dr. J. Richardson, Consultant specializing in pain management, for the care and concern shown to me;

Ruth Shaw, Chairperson of the Fibromyalgia Support and Carers' Group (West Yorkshire), and all the people like her who strive against their own ill health to raise fibromyalgia awareness and educate and support their fellow sufferers—I would, on behalf of all fibromyalgics, like to say that their efforts are truly appreciated;

Sharon Stephenson, Vice Chairperson of the Fibromyalgia Support and Carers' Group (West Yorkshire), for the time and effort she devotes to informing fibromyalgics and helping to run the group;

Bob Stewart, Chairperson of the Fibromyalgia Association UK, for all he continues to do for the Association and helping to bring fibromyalgia out from under its rock; and

Steve Taylor, a nutritionist, who has been a terrific help to me during the writing of this book. Steve has been with me every step of the way, providing valuable information and thoroughly checking my facts.

Foreword

Fibromyalgia syndrome (FMS) is a condition often misunderstood, or even disbelieved, by many in the medical profession. This reflects an unfortunate lack of knowledge, and the consequent frustration of doctors trained to cure recognized disease. The cause of FMS is unknown, and therefore treatment can be hampered in a traditional medical setting. It may help sufferers to know that lack of medical direction also suggests that FMS is not considered medically serious—it is not life threatening—but it is, of course, serious to the sufferer.

Treatment of FMS can, however, come from a different direction by focusing on and alleviating its effects on quality of life, rather than concentrating on finding a cause and cure. This approach is promoted throughout the book by strategies of self-management.

The book, then, is written for FMS sufferers. It reports on scientific findings and on a broad range of tried treatments. Interpretation of scientific findings is not yet conclusive and most treatments are made without the support of controlled studies. Nevertheless, exciting developments in areas such as functional brain imaging are followed with interest. The findings demonstrate a physiological basis for the pain of fibromyalgia, and also support cognitive behavioral therapy as the most effective management for the condition. Indeed, the book's emphasis on self-management is allied to such an approach.

Writing a book is an enormous achievement for someone suffering with FMS, and I implore sufferers and their carers to digest the contents of this one. If sufferers are enabled to develop better self-management and coping strategies through reading the book then Christine Craggs-Hinton has made a great contribution to the lives of those with this distressing condition.

If readers find that the principles of self-management make sense, but cannot execute the strategies in practice, they are more than halfway there. They can then join a group cognitive behavioral therapy program—often run by their regional rheumatology or pain clinic—to help in furthering their own self-management.

Jon Raphael, M.D.
Dudley Multidisciplinary Center
for Pain Management

Introduction

Fibromyalgia Syndrome (FMS) is a complicated condition, comprising a whole plethora of symptoms, including:

- fatigue
- stiffness
- migraines
- irritable bladder
- depression
- dry eyes
- insomnia
- anxiety
- irritable bowel syndrome
- allergies
- cold intolerance
- numbness

The chief characteristic, though, is that of chronic, widespread soft tissue pain, the intensity of which confounded medical professionals for many years.

Until recently fibromyalgics were told they either had arthritis (despite the absence of joint inflammation) or were suffering from psychological problems. Fortunately, the medical world is now slowly acknowledging the existence of fibromyalgia. Currently, more and more people are being diagnosed every day—and this comes as a great relief. To be told there is a real physical reason for the persistent pain and miscellany of additional symptoms is very heartening. Prior to diagnosis, many sufferers worry that their problems are of the mind rather than the body as tests have invariably proven negative, and family and friends, running short on patience, may even have begun urging, "Try to pull yourself together!" Other sufferers may have been convinced they were stricken with a terrible degenerative disease that, if not proving fatal, will eventually render them unable to function.

A fibromyalgic myself, I remember well the feelings of relief I experienced at my own diagnosis. It seemed like I had finally come to the end of a long journey that had begun eight years earlier with a whiplash injury. Now that my doctors knew what ailed me, I assumed they would immediately prescribe the appropriate medication. Before I knew it, I'd be back on my feet! I couldn't have been more wrong. I soon learned there are pills that lessen the symptoms, pills that make life a little more tolerable, but, sadly, no quick and simple cure-all.

Using the guidelines set out in Part One of this book, I was able to make vast improvements to my own condition. After being bed-bound and in terrible pain for several years, I found that gentle exercise, wiser use of medication, certain complementary therapies and pain and stress management techniques set me on the road to better health. I felt I was getting my life back—a different life than before my illness, I admit, but one in which real hope was beginning to flourish for the first time in years. I became able to manage my reduced levels of pain, accept my limitations and even to find the confidence to take on new challenges, such as writing this book. At the same time, I was not happy to stay as I was. That there was more help for me and my fellow fibromyalgics out there somewhere was something I was sure of—I just had to keep searching until I found it.

At one of my local fibromyalgia support group meetings, we were introduced to a Steve Taylor, a nutritionist. Steve—an enthusiastic, knowledgeable young man—informed us that it is possible to redress the many bodily imbalances in fibromyalgia by following a particular diet. He said it was possible for us to heal ourselves, using food. I knew instantly that this was what I had been searching for, so wasted no time in making the recommended improvements to my diet.

The "fibromyalgia healing diet" set out in Part Two of this book has become the most effective treatment I could have wished for—the foods used being, overall, no more expensive than the foods I was used to. I learned how to resolve the many nutritional deficiencies found in fibromyalgia; I learned about the toxic build-up caused, among other things, by food additives and preservatives; I learned how to follow a detoxification program to eliminate these toxins from my body, and many more things. It is not a calorie-counting diet, and I was relieved to find there are usually appetizing substitute foods that I can eat in place of those that have to be eliminated. It is largely a matter of checking labels at the supermarket and stopping off occasionally at the local health food store.

I soon found I was enjoying my new regime, making sure to maximize its effects by getting exercise and a little fresh air every day. More exciting, however, was the fact that, after a couple of months, my irritable bowel syndrome started to settle down, my pain levels were dropping sharply, and I had more energy than I had had in years. The other symptoms tied in with my fibromyalgia were becoming less of a problem, too—and all because of my changed diet!

Our bodies are powerful self-generating organisms. When provided with the right fuels, they start to heal themselves. This book sets out the recommended foods and nutritional supplements, as well as the substances to avoid and a 21-day detoxification program. The fibromyalgia healing diet stimulates healing of all the body's systems, allowing those systems to function in the way they were intended.

As I continue to eat the right foods and take the recommended nutritional supplements, I continue to improve. I cannot begin to describe how it feels to be so much better. It feels like I have been given a second chance at my life. I have to build up my strength now, quite substantially, by exercising, but, to be able to exercise and not feel shattered and in pain afterwards is wonderful in itself.

Admittedly, my life is still limited, and I have to remember to always pace myself. I still have days when I feel like caving in under the pressure of it all, but I am winning the battle. You can win, too. Just keep one thing in mind. You will have bad days, days when you may wonder "Is it all worth it?," but don't ever lose sight of the fact that once you have taken charge, once you have begun to arm yourself with knowledge—and with the impetus that brings—your condition will, in all probability, never be as bad as it was beforehand.

I must stress here that just as no two people with fibromyalgia suffer identical symptoms, so no two people will respond in the same way to the recommendations in this book. Some of you may find that in time your symptoms disappear completely; others may experience a less dramatic effect. However, I can assure you that there *will* be a change in your condition for the better, and that it will be at a fundamental level, for the recommendations in this book treat the *cause* of the disease, not just the *symptoms*.

Before You Start

The diet described in this book should only be followed with your doctor's approval. I am not able to independently dispense medical advice, nor can I prescribe remedies or assume any responsibility for those who treat themselves without the consent of their doctor. As some nutritional supplements may interact with certain medications and as they may adversely affect particular medical conditions, please consult your doctor before embarking on a course.

PART I

Living with Fibromyalgia

1

Fibro What?

*To be in constant pain, to feel too sapped to lift a limb, and to be
bombarded, at the same time, by a whole host of other ailments . . .
that's fibromyalgia!*

Although we are learning more and more about the causes of fibromyalgia syndrome (FMS for short), it remains a difficult condition to
diagnose. No one can see the pain, and it doesn't show itself in X-rays
or available blood tests and bone scans. You may have undergone a
whole gamut of "investigations," and while it is reassuring when major
illnesses are ruled out, you have probably prayed, at the same time, for
something to show up.

It may help to know that, prior to diagnosis, your doctor, likely as
not, felt as mystified as you. Ironically, your doctors' inability to determine the cause of your symptoms may be hampered by their medical
training. Medical students learn that specific conditions produce dis-
tinctive symptoms and that elimination of the cause ensures, in most
cases, full recovery. This "classical medical model" has been used successfully for many years, leading to numerous advances in modern
medicine. Unfortunately, because the difficulties fibromyalgia patients
present do not fit this model, delayed diagnosis is common.

On a more positive note, doctors are slowly but surely familiarizing
themselves with the peculiar nature of fibromyalgia. Research is making advances, too. Currently it is focusing on changes detected within

the central nervous system of sufferers. As is always the case when research takes a step toward solving the mystery of an illness, there is much optimism that advances in effective treatments will ensue.

What Is Fibromyalgia?

You may wonder how the name "fibromyalgia" came into being. The word can be split into parts that are easier to understand. "Fibro" means fibrous tissue—tendons and ligaments—"my" means muscle, and "algia" means pain. The word "syndrome" means a collection of symptoms that, when they occur together, identify an illness. The symptoms commonly occurring with fibromyalgia include persistent, widespread pain, fatigue, sleep disturbance, anxiety, irritable bowel problems, irritable bladder problems, reactive depression, headaches, allergies, "foggy brain" and morning stiffness (see Chapter 2).

Anyway . . . the good news first. Fibromyalgia is not a degenerative disease, it does not cause deformity and you will not die from it. Studies have shown that the majority of sufferers either stay the same or improve—and, although progress is generally slow, the changes can be dramatic. However, notable advances appear to be made only in those who take steps to help themselves.

Fibromyalgia is, without doubt, a "challenging" condition, for, as well as being incurable, its chief characteristic is pain. Sufferers often complain that they "hurt all over," although the neck, shoulders—generally in the region between the shoulder blades—chest, lower back and buttocks seem to be the principal areas affected. The pain is mainly muscular, but the tendons and ligaments are often involved. Due to nearby tense and painful tissues, joint mobility is occasionally reduced, too. There is no solid evidence to suggest that the joints sustain damage, however.

Widespread pain

The pain of fibromyalgia is commonly described as "widespread," and generally arises at neuromuscular junctions—that is, the places where the muscles receive electrical input from the nerve endings. Several areas may hurt at one time, but one particular region may be the cause of most concern. Also, the pain can migrate from area to area. One day your neck may hurt so badly you can barely turn your head; the next, although your neck has mysteriously eased, your legs ache so much that walking is difficult.

Such bizarre comings and goings of pain are difficult to rationalize, almost impossible for onlookers to comprehend and incredibly frustrating. Besides being random, the pain often fluctuates during the course of each day. Factors particular to each person can be responsible for aggravating it.

Stress is one of the greatest enemies of the fibromyalgia sufferer, as is the lack of restorative sleep, cold and/or humid weather conditions and too much or the wrong type of activity. Any one of these elements may provoke a flare-up of symptoms lasting for days, weeks or even months. On the other hand, sufferers may improve for no apparent reason.

Just as no two people are exactly alike, no two fibromyalgics experience precisely the same pain. One person may complain of searing, burning pains, another of throbbing sensations, another of tingling and numbness, and another of constant, nagging aches. Whatever the sensation felt, it is far from pleasant, and when accompanied by a multitude of other symptoms and illnesses, it is no wonder sufferers can be overwhelmed.

Pain origins

Pain from the following sources contributes to the overall picture.

- *Pain from muscle tension*   Muscle tension creates an increased demand for blood and oxygen, yet inhibits the drainage of waste materials. This creates more pain, therefore more muscle tension.
- *Pain from low muscle endurance*   Sustained activity creates many difficulties in fibromyalgia. For example, you may be able to lift, in turn, three two-pound bags of sugar without immediate pain, but shortly afterwards your muscles may begin to hurt. Lifting two bags of sugar would, in this instance, be recommended.
- *Myofascial (localized) pain*   This, often very acute, pain is induced by "trigger points" that are regularly "activated."
- *Pain from microtraumas*   Microtraumas are slow-healing microscopic tears in the muscle tissue. Experts believe they occur in most cases of fibromyalgia.

- *Pain from abnormal stiffness*   Extreme stiffness occurs frequently in fibromyalgia. It can arise when the individual sits or lies down for periods of time.

PAIN FROM MUSCLE TENSION

In all fibromyalgia sufferers, certain muscle groups are permanently tense and therefore painful. The tension may be due to overactivity, emotional stress or postural problems. Permanently tense muscles demand increased blood and oxygen supplies, but, at the same time, the muscle tension inhibits the drainage of waste materials. This leads to further tension and so further pain. The muscles eventually adapt to this cycle by becoming shorter and more fibrous, like the stringy bits in a piece of tough meat.

Gradually, these shorter, less elastic muscles begin to pull on their tendons—the structures that anchor them to the bones. The tendons then start the same process. Soon they, too, become deprived of oxygen; soon they, too, become clogged with waste materials. Like the affected muscles, they, in turn, grow fibrous and painful. Painful tissues burn energy at a terrific rate.

The tense and fibrous muscles go on to cause further problems, because for every set of tense muscles, there is an opposing set of weak muscles. For example, a person with weak abdominal muscles invari-

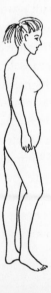

FIGURE 1   *Postural changes typical of fibromyalgia*

ably has tight lower back muscles. In the same way, each set of permanently tense and fibrous muscles has an opposite set of muscles that is permanently weakened. This eventually leads to the postural changes that typify fibromyalgia (*see Figure 1*).

TRIGGER POINTS

Not to be confused with the "tender points" used to diagnose fibromyalgia, trigger points are localized areas of pain and sensitivity occurring in permanently tense and fibrous tissues. Due to inadequate local circulation, these areas suffer from increased energy consumption and reduced oxygen supply.

When pressed, a trigger point will radiate pain and/or numbness into other areas. When "activated" by cold, stress, overexertion and so on, a trigger point will automatically transmit pain and numbness elsewhere. If your doctor pressed a certain point on your upper back, say, and as a result, you felt pain or numbness down one arm, the spot he had pressed would have been a trigger point.

Light-pressure trigger point massage generally reduces the pain and relaxes the muscle. (Pressure applied to tender points, on the other hand, will only increase overall pain.) Pain from active trigger points is a feature of almost all chronic pain conditions.

MYOFASCIAL PAIN SYNDROME

You may be surprised to learn that many fibromyalgics have myofascial pain syndrome (MPS for short), too. MPS arises from referred trigger point pain, which occurs when one or more trigger points are regularly "activated." It causes the localized, and often very severe, pain that is usually the worst part of our fibromyalgia. My myofascial pain is in my neck and upper back. Other common areas are the chest, buttocks and lower back.

MPS is diagnosed in the same way as fibromyalgia. The following four points, taken together, can indicate the existence of MPS:
1. the presence of chronic, localized pain;
2. the fact that there is no obvious cause of the pain—that is, joint strain or arthritis;
3. the fact that the pain has neither responded to treatments prescribed for what was originally thought to be the problem, nor to further treatments, including rest;

4. the fact that the pain intensifies when you are under different kinds of stress, such as after physical activity, emotional stress or exposure to cold.

There are some people, however, who have MPS without the presence of fibromyalgia. These people experience less morning stiffness, less fatigue and less incidence of digestive disorders. The best treatment of MPS is trigger point massage and manipulation—although, unfortunately, there are, to date, few physiotherapists trained in trigger point manipulation. On a short-term basis, trigger points respond well to heat treatments and acupuncture.

What Causes Fibromyalgia?

In fibromyalgia, the following abnormalities have been found in the processes and functions within the body and its various organs.

- *The central nervous system (brain and spinal cord)*   Advanced scanning technology has shown that people with fibromyalgia have reduced blood flow and energy production in the regions of the brain dealing with pain regulation, memory and concentration.
- *The endocrine system (hormones)*   Research into the endocrine system has shown that hormonal imbalances play a leading role in fibromyalgia. Research is now focusing on hormonal neurotransmitters.
- *The immune system (antibody protection against infection)*   Immune system disturbances resulting from an overload of environmental toxins (pesticides, aerosols, car fumes and so on) or viral activity can arise when activated by specific triggers.

Unfortunately, not enough is yet known about which abnormalities are most relevant to which particular symptom(s) occurring in fibromyalgia.

Chronic pain development

Physical trauma to virtually any area can progress into a chronic pain situation, and thereafter into fibromyalgia. The question of exactly how chronic pain arises has engendered much research into the pain processes and we are now considerably more enlightened. For many years, it was supposed that the same pain stimulus (that is, a pinprick) produced the same degree of pain. However, research has now proved that repetitious nerve stimulation causes an *amplification* of perceived pain.

Many experts believe that sensitization of the central nervous system (CNS)—that is, "central sensitization"—is the root cause of fibromyalgia. (The primary function of the CNS is to analyze input from nerve cells.) The first step toward central sensitization is the presence of persistent pain above a certain intensity. In 1992, researchers[1] found that persistent severe pain will only arise in individuals who have suffered severe pain in the past (the CNS "remembers" past pain intensity) and only after trauma, such as an injury or surgery, when the person concerned limits movement of the affected area. Given such circumstances, the individual is often dismayed to find that the pain has actually increased, rather than the reverse. That is how persistent pain can arise.

Persistent pain can quite easily advance into a chronic pain situation—the second step toward central sensitization. Modern scanning technology has demonstrated that enduring pain can create a gradual buildup of electrical response throughout the CNS. The currents can build to such an intensity that a state of chronic pain results, causing the CNS to become sensitized to pain. All chronic pain conditions involve a degree of central sensitization. Some sufferers are affected so severely they experience excruciating pain when performing the simplest of activities.

Neck trauma

Research conducted in 1997[2] suggests that physical trauma to the neck area is associated with a high risk of developing fibromyalgia. Dr. Buskila compared the progress of patients with soft-tissue neck injuries (usually occurring after whiplash) with patients suffering leg fractures. After approximately three months, he found that fibromyalgia is thirteen times more likely to develop following a neck injury than a lower extremity injury.

The difference may be due to the fact that the area injured in whiplash (the dorsal horn) plays an important role in filtering pain signals to the brain. Some experts believe that trauma to this area can severely impair the filtering mechanisms, allowing the pain-processing centers in the CNS to be bombarded with pain messages. They are of the opinion that such localized post-traumatic malfunction can gradually evolve into the widespread pain disorder that is fibromyalgia. As a result, many researchers are focusing on the pain-filtering mechanisms within the dorsal horn.

Spinal abnormalities

At the 1997 FMS International Conference Professor W. Muller presented a study that suggested that some fibromyalgics have structural abnormalities, occurring mostly in the cervical (neck) and lumbar (lower back) regions. Further studies using MRI (Magnetic Resonance Imaging) scans have shown a higher than normal incidence of narrowing of the spinal canal in the cervical region of some sufferers. The malformation is known as cervical stenosis and is usually genetic in origin. Experts are theorizing that mechanical irritations caused by spinal abnormalities can cause constant "injury" input to the CNS—effectively leading to sustained pain and central sensitization.

When the cervical spine is narrower than normal, tilting the neck backward can lead to spinal cord compression, which, in turn, restricts the flow of blood and spinal fluid to the CNS. Flexing the head forward, so your chin is near your chest, can stretch the spinal cord, causing mechanical irritation of the nerves running along it. This irritation is ultimately perceived as pain.

As most fibromyalgics suffer neck pain, activities that repeatedly flex the neck should be avoided. Instead of straining your neck, use your eyes more. Wearing a surgical collar will only weaken your muscles, and the likelihood of strain will increase once the collar is removed. Ultimately, strengthening your neck muscles by means of the exercises described in Chapter 4 is the most useful advice I can offer.

Abnormal hormone levels

Medical professionals have long been bewildered by the severity of pain in fibromyalgia. Recent studies have shown, however, due in part to the effects of central sensitization—very low pain thresholds—that fibromyalgics have. A sufferer may feel distinct and troublesome pain where a healthy person may only feel discomfort. This in no way signifies that sufferers are "soft" or "weak," for evidence suggests that fibromyalgics actually complain far less than the average person.

The pain of fibromyalgia not only comes from a variety of sources, it can also be provoked and amplified by abnormalities in certain body chemicals. We now know that elevated levels of the pain-transmitting chemical substance P is one of the principal causes of severe pain in fibromyalgia, whereas low levels of the chemical serotonin may be primarily responsible for the lack of pain control.

Substance P plays an important role in the biochemical pain sequence. When a person experiences a painful trauma, such as a smashed finger, there is an immediate release of substance P into the spinal cord. A series of messages are then transmitted, one of which tells the brain that the finger is injured. Several studies have shown that, regardless of the triggering factor in fibromyalgia, the level of substance P present in the spinal fluid is elevated to three times that of healthy people. This indicates that fibromyalgics experience a greater level of perceived pain than normal. Other chronic pain disorders display slight elevations of substance P, but the levels are not nearly so high as in fibromyalgia.

As mentioned, chronic pain can give rise to central sensitization. Fibromyalgia apparently arises when pain-transmitting chemicals—the primary one being substance P—accumulate to such an extent that they overflow from injured tissues to neighboring healthy tissues, increasing their sensitivity to pain. In some instances, this hormone can pervade the entire spinal cord. As a consequence, everyday activity can result in pain that, in turn, can lead to impaired function. Indeed, sensitization of erstwhile healthy tissues may even cause light touch to be experienced as pain. After doing something as seemingly insignificant as scratching a tiny itch, many fibromyalgics—myself included—experience acute pain in that area lasting several minutes.

Pain circuitry

Although an excess of substance P is perhaps the primary cause of the sustained pain of fibromyalgia, research[3] conducted in 1991 suggests that altered neuron programming can add to the problem. There are two types of nerve fibers—nociceptive neurons and non-nociceptive neurons—multitudes of which exist alongside each other throughout the body. Normally, an injury such as a smashed finger produces distinct physical and chemical changes that are picked up by nociceptive neurons. Messages, one of which creates the consciousness of localized pain, are rapidly relayed between the finger and the CNS. (The same series of events takes place with all peripheral injuries—a broken arm, cut knee, stubbed toe or whatever.) The non-nociceptive nerve fibers in the injured area are not normally involved in the pain process. These fibers relay only tactile-type messages to the CNS. Such messages usually involve sensations of touch—a kiss, stroke, pat on the back or light massage. They also transmit sensations of muscle movement—walking, raising your arms or turning your head.

However, when the CNS is hypersensitized, previously innocuous non-nociceptive neurons can be hijacked into becoming pain transmitters. Dr. Woolf has, in fact, been able to show that, in chronic pain conditions, non-nociceptive neurons can alter their programming to mimic nociceptive neurons. Some are such mimics they even start releasing substance P—another reason that fibromyalgics encounter pain during experiences that are not ordinarily painful.

It must be stated that not all chronic pain conditions hijack non-nociceptive neurons into acting as pain messengers. We can only assume that a person's genetic make-up determines whether or not they will be affected.

Familial links

Research indicates that fibromyalgia can run in families. This may be due to the shared family environment (exposure to the same oil/gas fumes, aerosol sprays, glue, varnish and so on), or it may be genetic in nature. In some cases, it may even be both. Preliminary evidence suggests that the condition can indeed be inherited, particularly by the women in a family. Men have the same family genes, but their hormonal milieu appears to offer a measure of protection.

Who Gets Fibromyalgia?

Anyone can develop fibromyalgia, but, probably due to hormonal differences, it is present in roughly seven times more women than men. The onset of the condition is usually between the ages of 25 and 50, although many children are affected, and it can arise in people aged 75

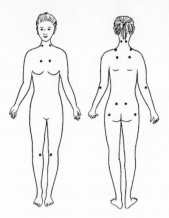

FIGURE 2 *The 18 tender points used to establish a diagnosis of fibromyalgia*

and over. Fibromyalgia is very common, too. Surveys in various countries point to it affecting up to 3.2 percent of the population, and numerous cases have not yet been diagnosed. As the symptoms of fibromyalgia vary so much in severity, some experts believe many sufferers have either not yet consulted a doctor or have had their health problems dismissed as anxiety, depression, neurosis and such or as symptoms of another disorder from which they are known to be suffering.

Diagnosis

Fibromyalgics have areas of tenderness in specific locations—usually at junctions of muscle and bone. These areas are known as tender points. They may be exquisitely painful when pressed. Otherwise they may or may not cause pain.

In 1990, the American College of Rheumatology defined the official criteria for the diagnosis of fibromyalgia:
- a history of pain in both sides of the body, pain above and below the waist, pain along the spine; and
- pain or tenderness in 11 out of 18 tender points, sited at specific locations in the body (*see Figure 2*).

Treatment

Doctors are trained to strive to cure illness. The gratification they experience from restoring patients to full health makes their job worthwhile.

It is usually the reason they entered the medical profession in the first place. In fact, we visit them because we expect to be offered a cure. So what happens when patients are diagnosed with fibromyalgia, for which currently there is no cure?

Unfortunately, there is little doctors can do to correct the disorders underlying fibromyalgia. Painkillers can reduce pain for a time, they may prove invaluable in a flare-up, but they have no positive long-term effects. Certain antidepressants are known to go some way toward redressing the chemical imbalance of fibromyalgia, but they are unable to permanently correct it. Patients may even suffer adverse side effects after taking medications for a long period. Referrals to physical therapy are also commonplace in fibromyalgia. However, as physical therapists may know little or nothing of the condition, manipulation and prescribed exercise can aggravate the pain. The doctor may later refer the patient to relevant specialists dealing with the disorders connected with fibromyalgia—a gastroenterologist if irritable bowel syndrome is diagnosed or an allergy clinic if allergies are an issue. Treatments for these conditions may prove beneficial, but such people can do little to minimize the main symptom—pain.

Some doctors may choose to make referrals to pain or rheumatology clinics, but, again, the patient is invariably disappointed. Assessments are all too brief and although some patients may be offered painkilling injections, they are not suitable for everyone. The majority of sufferers are dismissed feeling they haven't been taken seriously. It may help to know that what appears to be disinterest is, in many cases, sheer frustration at being unable to do or say anything useful. Fibromyalgia is an illness that is best helped by emotional guidance, and all forms of self-help should be encouraged.

It is a fact that because nothing further can be done at pain or rheumatology clinics, fibromyalgia patients are swiftly discharged. For a long time this circumstance led to an unfortunate misconception that prevented the condition being given due respect. Hospital managers, statisticians, researchers and the like assumed fibromyalgia patients were discharged because they had improved so much they no longer needed help. This error was only recently spotted.

For many years, chronic, intractable pain has presented a stumbling block for doctors. They have long recognized that "temporary" treatments are not the answer, but apart from referring patients to a pain clinic or rheumatologist for what they know will be a brief period, there has been little else they can do. There is hope, however. At last many health authorities are recognizing the need to adopt a different approach for chronic pain patients who accept that there is no available cure for their condition.

Primary care rehabilitation programs are employing a multidimensional approach to the physical and psychosocial problems that arise with chronic pain. This involves teaching the patient a variety of pain management techniques, as well as a paced physical activity program. Pain rehabilitation programs do not offer a cure, but they can mean that the patient understands more about the nature of chronic pain and is more physically active, less emotionally distressed, able to use a range of relaxation skills and, ultimately, less reliant on medication. A pain sufferer who attended one hospital's first program is noted as saying, "From the beginning I realized they were just like me, frustrated and in pain—and from all walks of life. We were not promised a cure, but we were going to learn how to manage our pain."

2

All Part of the Syndrome

I thought I was going out of my mind! Sleep problems, stomach problems,
fatigue, a sensitivity to many of the everyday things in life—
on top of the constant pain . . . It was such a relief to find
they were all part of the same illness!

Fibromyalgia, as we have seen, is a syndrome, which means that several conditions are commonly associated with the disorder. These conditions may be present without fibromyalgia, but they are so often seen with fibromyalgia that they are now considered a part of the syndrome. This chapter deals with the most common of these conditions, excluding muscle pain, which is discussed in other chapters.

Conditions commonly occurring with fibromyalgia are:

- muscular pain
- disturbed sleep
- anxiety
- headaches
- muscle spasms
- morning stiffness
- irritable bladder
- skin problems
- fatigue
- depression
- irritable bowel syndrome
- allergies
- cognitive dysfunction ("foggy brain")
- dry eyes and mouth
- restless arms and legs
- numbness and tingling
- temporomandibular joint dysfunction (jaw pain)

Other possible symptoms are:

- bloated feeling (particularly in hands and feet)
- photophobia (extreme sensitivity to light)
- chronic rhinitis (a persistently runny nose)
- bruxism (teeth grinding during sleep)
- mouth ulcers
- bruising easily

Fatigue

Chronic fatigue is virtually universal in fibromyalgia. In some it is barely discernible, but in others it is extreme, like the exhaustion that comes with a bad dose of flu. At times, your muscles may feel worn to their limit, even though you have just woken up. People less severely affected may find that relaxing in a chair for half an hour is enough to restore their flagging energy levels.

The best way to manage all but extreme weariness is to alternate activity with periods of rest. The key is to listen to your body. Don't try to push yourself when you feel exhausted already. Finishing off that pile of ironing before you flop onto the sofa will only make you feel worse.

Serotonin

Most fibromyalgics are known to have an abnormally low supply of serotonin—a neurotransmitter that sends messages to the vital organs via the blood chemistry. Serotonin interacts with substance P to determine pain levels. Medication that helps slow down the removal of serotonin (selective serotonin re-uptake inhibitors, or SSRIs) can help combat fatigue, depression, sleep problems and so on. Such drugs include paroxetine (Paxil), sertraline (Zoloft) and fluoxetine (Prozac).

Seasonal affective disorder (SAD)

During winter, the decline in daylight hours can cause a marked deficiency in serotonin availability, triggering an increase in fatigue, depression, anxiety and so on in susceptible people. This phenomenon gives rise to what is now known as seasonal affective disorder (SAD), which affects many people each winter.

As people with fibromyalgia have serotonin in low supply anyway, it explains, in part, why their symptoms generally worsen in winter. Treatment to replace the availability of serotonin can take the form of light therapy—that is, exposure for up to four hours a day to very bright light, at least 10 times the intensity of ordinary domestic lighting. The individual should sit 2 to 3 feet from a specially designed lightbox, placed perhaps on a table, where they can then carry out normal activities—reading, writing, eating, knitting and so on. Provided the lightbox is used daily, benefits should be felt within three or four days and will continue throughout the winter months.

When fibromyalgia sufferers use light therapy in conjunction with medication that moderates the removal of serotonin (SSRIs), the difficulties encountered during the winter months can be greatly reduced.

Hypoglycemia

A word or two of warning. Fatigue should never be presumed to be an element of fibromyalgia. Your particular symptoms may relate to any one of numerous disorders, so they should always be discussed with your doctor. For example, headaches, confusion, visual disturbance, muscle weakness, impaired muscle coordination and extreme mood swings should all be taken seriously as indications of a type of hypoglycemia. Another type of hypoglycemia is characterized by faintness, weakness, jitteriness, nervousness and excessive hunger.

Early diagnosis of hypoglycemia is crucial. (If left untreated, the first set of symptoms can lead to loss of consciousness, convulsions and, eventually, coma.)

Myalgic encephalomyelitis (ME)

In discussing fatigue, myalgic encephalomyelitis (ME for short) should be mentioned, as, for several years, many medical professionals have been of the opinion that fibromyalgia and ME (also known as chronic fatigue syndrome, or CFS for short) are different strains of the same illness. The two do indeed have many symptoms in common, but experts now assure us that each is in fact a distinct syndrome in its own right.

Sleep Problems

As with muscle pain and fatigue, sleep problems appear to be present in all cases of fibromyalgia. In fact, poor sleep quality is seen as being a cause of the condition as well as a result. Due to the abnormal brain wave patterns known to be found in fibromyalgics, most are simply unable to achieve deep, restorative sleep.

Throughout sleep, the brain continues to rule the body functions by controlling the release of various hormones. The levels of prolactin and testosterone—the growth hormones—rise significantly during deep, delta-phase sleep, facilitating tissue repair and regeneration. Good health depends on an individual being able to achieve this type of restorative sleep each and every night. Wouldn't you just know it, the majority of fibromyalgics have difficulty attaining delta-phase sleep. Light, alpha-phase sleep constantly interrupts this important level, causing the person to wake feeling almost as tired as when they retired the previous night.

Because delta-phase sleep is rarely achieved in fibromyalgia, most sufferers find their growth hormones are in low supply. These essential hormones can, to some extent, be induced by changing to a high-protein diet, taking mineral supplements—preferably before bedtime—and using relaxation techniques. However, if a fibromyalgic takes no action to replace at least some of the lost growth hormones, the lack of delta-phase sleep can cause the muscles to continue to suffer.

In 1993, a researcher[4] was able to demonstrate how easily disturbed sleep can affect the muscles. Six volunteers (people without fibromyalgia) were repeatedly woken during delta-phase sleep for three consecutive nights; they all began to display the diffuse pain, fatigue and tender sites present in fibromyalgia. On the other hand, fully fit long-distance runners were unaffected after being disturbed in the same way. It can be seen, therefore, that carefully controlled lifestyle changes, involving dietary improvements, better relaxation and the careful introduction of exercise can be very helpful to fibromyalgia sufferers.

Depression and Anxiety

Depression, as you can imagine, is commonly found in chronic pain sufferers. Wouldn't anyone become depressed if they had pain every day? Until fairly recently, depression was believed to be one of the factors leading to the development of fibromyalgia. Nowadays, it is recognized as being a *reaction* to the condition.

One of the most unfortunate features of fibromyalgia is its invisibility. No one can see the pain, and people tend to look blank, maybe even suspicious, when you explain that you suffer from fibromyalgia. "Fibro what?" They have never heard of it! "Does it mean you ache a bit from time to time? We all ache a bit! Surely you're just being oversensitive!" This type of reaction really can trigger mild depression or emphasize that which is already present. It is advisable to concentrate on the people in your life who at least try to understand how you feel. Doing so can eliminate many negative feelings.

Anxiety is widespread among fibromyalgics. As with depression, anxiety often arises as a result of being in pain constantly tired and from an endless barrage of other unpleasant symptoms. Fibromyalgics who have no choice but to limit certain activities often become anxious prior to attempting something unfamiliar. The more insular the individual has become, the more difficult out-of-the-ordinary situations are for them to handle.

To determine anxiety, ask yourself these questions.

- Am I more easily upset than usual?
- Do I feel I am overreacting to certain situations?
- Am I unusually edgy?
- Do I find it difficult to relax?
- Am I having more than usual trouble sleeping?
- Am I breathing more shallowly than usual?

If you can answer "yes" to any one of these questions, you are probably suffering from anxiety. Anxiety has the effect of stimulating the sympathetic nervous system—the mechanisms in the brain that respond automatically to certain occurrences—making you more tense, more tired and ultimately more anxious. Learning to relax effectively is easier said than done, but as anxiety is such a distressing condition, it is worth trying to follow a regular deep breathing and relaxation routine.

Relaxed muscles use far less energy than tense ones, and improved breathing leads to better circulation and oxygenation, which in turn help the muscles and connective tissues. A calm, relaxed mind can greatly aid concentration and short-term memory. It can also clear brain fog.

To cope with anxiety more effectively, it is advisable to either limit or cut out certain stimulants, particularly caffeine, alcohol and tobacco.

Stimulants are known to exacerbate anxiety, and the aforementioned products are the chief culprits. In fact, most of the symptoms of chronic anxiety may be due to the effects of high intakes of caffeine alone.

Panic attacks

More commonly known as a panic attack, acute hyperventilation, or overbreathing, is a common affliction in fibromyalgia. A panic attack is an emotional response to anticipated stress. Often the perceived threat is obvious, but sometimes there are no apparent reasons for the onset of panicky feelings. In the latter instance, the reason may be buried in earlier life events. Talking to a counselor may unlock buried fears and help the individual see them in a new, more manageable light.

As a rule, panic attacks are preceded by intensifying anxiety. The individual will start breathing faster in troubled apprehension. Light-headedness, palpitations and the sensation that the chest is tightening will then be accompanied by feelings of inadequacy, fear and maybe of impending doom.

Daily deep breathing exercises—where breathing is slowed down and, on inhalation, the abdomen (not the ribcage) is allowed to rise—are very useful training. An immediate remedy is the good old paper bag. Place the paper bag over your nose and mouth and try to breathe more slowly. Breathing into the bag will ensure that most of the exhaled carbon dioxide is returned to your lungs. (Correct breathing is discussed in great detail in Chapter 6.)

Irritable Bowel Syndrome (IBS)

Fibromyalgia is, to a large extent, a problem of muscle irritability. This fact is more obvious in the muscles under voluntary control—those of the back, shoulders, stomach, buttocks and so on—but the so-called "smooth" muscles under involuntary control can be equally affected, giving rise to bowel and bladder problems as well as headaches.

Many experts believe that irritable bowel syndrome (IBS) arises largely as a result of muscle irritability. Fibromyalgia and IBS do appear to be closely linked. It appears that more than half of the people diagnosed with IBS display many of the symptoms of fibromyalgia.

IBS is characterized by recurrent cramping pains, together with alternating bouts of diarrhea and constipation, but some people have just diarrhea or just constipation. Abdominal gas, bloating, heartburn, backache, nausea and lethargy are all elements of the syndrome, too. The majority of people suffer from just a few of the above symptoms, but an unlucky minority are cursed with them all.

A survey conducted in 1997 by the Fibromyalgia Network, Arizona revealed that 64 percent of fibromyalgics suffer IBS.

Chronic yeast infections and IBS

IBS has no single, distinct cause, but research has shown that it can develop after a severe bout of gastroenteritis or after taking a course of antibiotics—prescribed, maybe, to treat the infection. Antibiotics effectively kill the microorganisms that cause disease, but they kill friendly bacteria at the same time, causing an imbalance of the intestinal microflora.

Friendly bacteria are essential to the well-being of the digestive system, for they not only aid digestion, they also protect against parasitic yeast infections, commonly known as thrush or candida (*candida albicans*). Indeed, candida infections were relatively unknown until the advent of antibiotics in the 1940s!

Although some practitioners remain skeptical about the role of candida in IBS, many others have found that when the infection is eliminated, the symptoms of IBS decrease. Candida growth may be encouraged by the Pill, steroids, immunosuppressive anti-inflammatory drugs, nutritional deficiencies, high-sugar diets and by any condition that weakens the immune system. Cancer and AIDS are obvious examples. (See page 155 for more information.)

Mercury fillings and IBS

There is a growing tide of feeling that the mercury used in dental fillings is at the root of many of today's illnesses. Some researchers are convinced that mercury leaking from amalgam fillings interferes with the immune system. They believe that instead of killing bad bacteria, the immune system, confused, begins to attack the body's own cells— the muscles and ligaments. In this situation, the immune system would then begin to set up antibodies to certain foods, thus developing food intolerance. Again we see a possible link between fibromyalgia and IBS.

Food intolerance and IBS

Whether or not there is a link between food intolerance and IBS has engendered much dispute in the medical world. Many natural practitioners believe food intolerance to be the underlying cause of IBS, while many conventional doctors reject the theory outright.

Such diverse opinion may arise in part because of confusion between the words "allergy" and "intolerance." When we discover that a certain food disagrees with us, we say we are "allergic" to it. However, as there is generally no immunological reaction to that food—that is, if our body fails to act as if it is being invaded by a foreign body, thereby setting up "antibody" chemicals—we are using the wrong term.

A true allergy produces anything from a runny nose, hives or a migraine attack to an extreme, life-threatening immune response such as anaphylactic shock. Intolerance, on the other hand, is caused by a slow buildup of "problem" foods and, unlike an allergic reaction where the backlash is immediate, the response is delayed. The body eventually becomes sensitized to foods—often, ironically, the ones we eat most—inducing anything from stomach irritation (abdominal cramps, perhaps accompanied by diarrhea), to cravings, to indigestion, all of which are unpleasant.

An increasing body of evidence is prompting experts to believe that IBS develops as a result of food intolerance. Sadly, it would appear that because many researchers fail to allow for the delayed response, the vital connection is missed.

The foods most likely to cause problems are wheat, corn, food colorings, coffee, yeasts, citrus fruits and dairy products, as well as foods containing chemical additives and preservatives (in effect, all processed foods). Food intolerance will always be a threat to people who fail to eat a varied diet. A safe and mild cleansing regime, where problem foods are excluded, then slowly re-introduced, can help reduce food intolerance.

Stress and IBS

Stress and anxiety are believed to contribute to the development of IBS and are known to play a major role in intensifying the symptoms. Stress can have the effect of suppressing the immune system, the employment of stress-relieving techniques is usually helpful in treating IBS.

Any out-of-the-ordinary bowel activity must be reported to your doctor. Depending on your particular symptoms, the doctor may decide to refer you to a specialist for tests. A diagnosis of IBS is normally made when symptoms persist and yet no specific bowel disorder is evident.

Headaches

As headaches are a common symptom of many of the conditions occurring with fibromyalgia, it is hardly surprising that, according to a 1998 survey[5], 59 percent of sufferers endure them regularly. Tension headaches and migraines are most prevalent. Sometimes, however, headaches can be provoked by a sinus infection. Your doctor should be informed of your exact symptoms.

Tension headaches

Less intense than a migraine, tension headaches are miserable nevertheless. Tension in the neck—from where the pain usually originates—causes muscles to contract, giving rise to the feeling of a tight elastic band across the affected area. Pain is often first felt at the base of the neck, spreading upward to the temples.

Painkillers are invaluable for all types of headaches, but they are most effective in the early stages of pain. However, as stress no doubt aggravates and may even be the cause of most headaches, it is useful to learn stress-management techniques. A simple tip—lavender essential oil, mixed as directed on the bottle with a carrier oil, massaged into the forehead and temples can help reduce the pain.

Migraine

This type of acutely painful headache is characterized by one-sided intense throbbing, sensitivity to light and sound, nausea and sometimes vomiting. Attacks are caused by the constriction and dilation of the tiny capillaries that take blood to the brain and can be triggered by stress, anxiety, fatigue, watching television, loud noises, flickering light and a sensitivity to such things as red wine, aged and strong cheeses, chocolate, coffee, tea, alcohol and cured meats such as hot dogs, salami, bacon and ham.

I recommended keeping a record each time of all the foods and drinks consumed in the hours preceding an attack. It should not take long for the trigger factors to become apparent.

Smokers who suffer regular migraine attacks would be wise to quit. Smokers typically have narrowed blood vessels anyway, so migraine attacks are always a possibility. Regular exercise is important (see Chapter 5), as is eating healthily. It is advisable to eat three or more small meals a day and never skip a meal. Helpful complementary therapies include homeopathy, herbal medicine, acupuncture, cranial osteopathy and reflexology.

Allergies

It is estimated that half the people with fibromyalgia also have a history of allergy (toxicity) problems. The allergenic substances may be environmental (dust or pollen) or a specific medication may be responsible. However, it is likely that some so-called "allergic" reactions are simply a part of the enhanced sensitivity that goes with fibromyalgia.

Chemical sensitivity

Some researchers are now of the opinion that exposure to certain chemicals in our environment (pesticides, artificial fertilizers, petrochemical fumes, glue, varnish, aerosol sprays, some household cleaners, some paints, some perfumes . . . the list is endless) as well as exposure to certain medications, may be responsible for many of the symptoms found in both fibromyalgia and ME. It is no coincidence that, with few exceptions, in countries with little industrial power and where fresh food is grown without chemicals and eaten straight from the land, there is generally a marked absence or low incidence of allergies.

Chemical sensitivity can give rise to profound effects, including fatigue, headaches, nausea, short-term memory loss, mood changes and numbness and tingling in the fingers and toes. A sensitivity to certain chemicals, on the other hand, is thought to restrict blood flow to and through the parts of the brain dealing with pain regulation, memory and concentration. Furthermore, a chemically overloaded immune system may, in its growing confusion, begin to react to all manner of environmental substances, and chemically sensitive individuals are more likely than others to develop true allergies.

Dr. Joe Fitzgibbon, in his 1993 book *Feeling Tired All the Time*, illustrates how grim chemical sensitivity can be. With chronic exposure to oil and later gas fumes, his wife developed intense migraine attacks, nausea, vomiting, extreme exhaustion and eventually, partial paralysis. She was ill for four years. Then, after staying with friends in an all-electric house for a while, the symptoms miraculously receded. Needless to say, the couple moved into an all-electric house of their own!

Sensitization to chronic chemical exposure is now well documented. Mechanics have been known to become sensitized to gasoline fumes, painters to paint, printers to ink and so on. Maybe we should all take a closer look at our immediate environments. Eliminating—or at least reducing—our particular trigger factors could greatly lessen some of the symptoms tied in with our fibromyalgia. Trigger factors are not always easy to spot, however. Many medical professionals maintain that a healthy diet, rest, relaxation and plenty of exercise can help increase the body's tolerance of chemicals.

Gulf War Syndrome

In the meantime, chemical sensitivity is being vigorously researched—particularly after the problems veterans of the first Gulf War have had as a result of the exposure to cocktails of chemicals during their tours of duty. It is interesting to note that Gulf War veterans afflicted with what is now called Gulf War Syndrome report precisely the same symptoms as do people with fibromyalgia.

Muscle Spasms

Muscle spasms are common in fibromyalgia, occurring most frequently in the back, buttocks and legs. They can be defined as involuntary muscular contractions and feel rather like the affected area is in cramp. The muscles contract due to reduced blood flow and a resulting shortage of oxygen to the muscle tissues.

Microtrauma

Muscle microtrauma (microscopic tears in the muscle fibers) may be an additional cause of spasms. For a few days after overexertion, these small tears can leak substances that cause muscle stiffness and pain. In addition, microtrauma is believed to reduce the production of energy in the muscle, thereby causing muscle fatigue.

Some experts believe that fibromyalgics have a great deal of muscle microtrauma, and that it occurs because of a genetic predisposition. The microtrauma can be limited by pacing yourself, increasing exercise levels at a very slow rate and stopping an activity as soon as your muscles begin to protest.

The use of cold rather than heat in treatment

Spasms can be prevented by regularly changing positions and keeping as mobile as possible. The pain of a spasm can be relieved by the use of heat, massage or gentle trigger point pressure.

Cold is an effective painkiller, too. The mere mention of the word "cold" may cause a person with fibromyalgia to wince. Cold weather can induce a severe flare-up, so how can it relax a muscle spasm? There is a great difference between walking to the store on a bitterly cold day and applying cold directly to trigger points or other tender areas. Ice helps numb the pain of a toothache or a sore finger; it helps relieve muscle pain in the same way. A bag of frozen peas is ideal for this purpose as it molds to the right shape, but remember to first wrap the bag in a cloth to protect the skin. A routine of 10 minutes on, then 10 minutes off, works best.

Cognitive Dysfunction ("Foggy Brain")

Short-term memory loss, word mixups, and difficulties with concentration are problems many fibromyalgics are familiar with. Cognitive dysfunction is usually attributed to the shortage of deep sleep and the fact that the individual's attention is often focused on trying to cope with the pain. The problem is also intensified by fatigue.

Studies have failed to indicate any functional abnormalities in the memory and thought processes, but modern scanning techniques have shown that fibromyalgics suffer from restricted blood flow to the parts of the brain controlling memory and concentration. The deep breathing and relaxation techniques outlined in Chapter 6 are excellent for improving the circulation to and through the brain. Hydrotherapy and stretching exercises aid circulation, too.

I suggest getting into the habit of writing things down, especially important dates and forthcoming events. Making lists may be tedious, but it is nice when you get to the store and know exactly why you went there! Personally, I have found my lists of "things to do" invaluable.

Morning Stiffness

Morning stiffness is common in fibromyalgia. It generally occurs after the individual has spent maybe several hours lying in one position—overnight, for example, hence the name. In some people the condition is severe and may arise after sitting for a short time. The stiffness can take three or four hours to wear off and so may discourage a person affected from taking bus or car trips or going to the movies, theater and so on.

Changing position regularly and moving around freely wherever possible does help. Walking around to avoid overnight stiffness is not practical, but getting into a hot bath or shower the first thing in the morning can minimize the discomfort. Regular morning muscle stretching exercises is helpful, too.

Irritable Bladder

Many people with fibromyalgia have the feeling that their bladder is full most of the time. Urination may be painful and so a urinary infection may be suspected. Tests, however, usually show no evidence of infection. The problem is solely muscle irritation. If you find you need to urinate frequently, see your doctor.

Dry Eyes and Mouth (Sicca Syndrome)

About a third of all fibromyalgics report dry eyes and dry mouth—"sicca" means dry. As the eyes may burn and itch, your doctor should be informed. Eye drops, applied twice daily, will help to prevent painful reddening.

A dry mouth is likely to be caused by medication; antidepressant medications are notorious for this. It is therefore advisable to check the side effects of your prescribed drugs. Sucking hard candy or chewing gum is helpful.

Restless Arms and Legs

Falling asleep is difficult enough for people with fibromyalgia. It can be distressing when, on top of that, your legs ache terribly, no matter how often you shift position. Then, when you have finally dropped off, you may be snapped awake by jerking limbs or the fierce gripping pain of a leg cramp. Not pleasant!

Restless leg syndrome

Restless leg syndrome is not uncommon in fibromyalgia. It is characterized by an intense feeling of restlessness in the legs, particularly when lying in bed, trying to get to sleep. Cramps, especially in the calf muscles, are also associated with this syndrome. Gentle movement—walking around—can give temporary relief.

Nocturnal myoclonus

Sudden involuntary spasms in the arms and legs during sleep may also be experienced by fibromyalgics. This is known as nocturnal myoclonus—"nocturnal" meaning nighttime, "myoclonus" meaning sudden contraction of the muscles. In severe cases, anti-spasmodic drugs may help. In mild to moderate cases, herbal remedies may prove beneficial.

Both of the above-mentioned sleep disorders can be frustrating for the sufferer, and, when limbs start flying, not exactly pleasant for the person sharing the bed either! They can also severely interfere with sleep and the body's ability to rejuvenate the cells, recharging the batteries. Many experts regard these disorders as being caffeine-related.

Numbness and Tingling (Paresthesia)

Paresthesia is the correct medical term for spontaneous burning, pricking, numbness or tingling—usually in the fingers and toes. When a doctor uses the term, it means that there is no obvious reason for the sensations, so further investigations need to be made.

When the underlying problem is fibromyalgia, it indicates that soft tissue problems (fibrotic muscles and so on) are interfering with the transmission of nerve messages. However, as with all the symptoms associated with fibromyalgia, they should never merely be assumed to be a part of the illness. Paresthesia may be a symptom of any one of several different conditions and should always be reported to your doctor.

Skin Problems

Many fibromyalgics have sensitive skins. If a sufferer is scratched so that a red mark appears, that mark will often linger for an unusually long time. This is particularly apparent in skin overlying the person's most painful regions, and is attributed to a hyperactive sympathetic nervous system. In other words, nerve messages are being inappropriately transmitted.

Irritations and rashes

Some fibromyalgics experience regular itching, and rashes may develop. Hot baths, warm clothing and mild stress may make the problem worse. Rashes should be treated by the application of calamine lotion or hydrocortisone cream. There is as yet no known cause, and treatment is not always successful.

Reynaud's phenomenon

Reynaud's phenomenon is an abnormal and exaggerated response to stimulation—cold or stress—that causes the blood vessels in the fingers or toes to narrow. The restricted blood flow then causes the affected areas to turn white or even bluish. The condition is almost always associated with disorders affecting the body's connective tissues—the blood vessels, skin, muscles, tendons and joints—and so is occasionally found in individuals with fibromyalgia.

People who smoke can limit the attacks by giving up the habit. Smoking tends to narrow the blood vessels anyway and so will only exacerbate the condition. Reynaud's patients would be well advised to avoid drugs that cause the blood vessels to narrow further. The list includes some varieties of the Pill and some heart, blood and migraine medications. It is important that individuals with this condition remember to keep warm.

Temporomandibular Joint Dysfunction (Jaw Pain)

Facial pain affects about a quarter of the fibromyalgia population. For some it is part of the diffuse pain that characterizes the condition, but for others it comes from a malfunction of the temporomandibular joint (TMJ), which links the upper and lower jaws. Tense and fibrotic muscles and ligaments provoke pain in front of the ear when chewing, usually accompanied by a cracking or crunching sound. There may also be difficulty opening the mouth. Other symptoms of TMJ dysfunction include headaches, facial numbness, dizziness and ringing in the ears.

The condition is commonly caused by traumatic impact, maybe as a result of a traffic accident, a fall, a blow or even dental work. Dentists should be the first port of call where treatment is concerned. They may refer you to a dental specialist; a specially made splint worn over the lower teeth can greatly improve the situation.

3

Medication

*At last I had a diagnosis; at last I understood that
my varied symptoms were all elements of one disease. "
So what can you do for me, doctor?" I asked. He pulled out
his prescription pad and began to write . . .*

The Need for Chemical Intervention

It is only natural that we look first to our doctors for help, and drugs
are, almost without exception, the first course of action for newly diagnosed fibromyalgics. Only later do we begin to look at other, more natural therapies that, unlike drugs, have neither side effects nor addictive
qualities. However, as most drugs have an almost immediate effect and
indisputably go a long way toward suppressing the pain of fibromyalgia, they usually continue to play an important role in managing the
condition, helping us live a more active, fulfilling life.

As fibromyalgics are often sensitive to medication, its benefits
should always be weighed against its side effects. Commencing a
course of medication on a very low dosage can markedly reduce its side
effects. Remember that no one type of medication works for everyone.
It is always wise to work closely with your doctor to find the drugs that
are most suitable for you.

Painkillers (Analgesics)

Painkillers are invaluable in fibromyalgia. Many doctors advise patients to take painkillers regularly, keeping the level in the blood more or less constant and thereby offering relief throughout the day. This works well for acute pain, such as that experienced during a flare-up, but, as prolonged, high-dosage painkiller usage can lead to a reduction in its effectiveness (a situation whereby the patient needs to take more and more to achieve the same result) as well as addiction and eventually stomach, liver and/or kidney problems, it is not such a good idea for the long term.

Over-the-counter painkillers

This category includes aspirin and acetaminophen medications, each of which are capable of keeping mild to moderate pain at bay. Inform your doctor of long-term over-the-counter drug usage. Enteric-coated pills are easier on the stomach.

Many over-the-counter creams and gels have a warming, soothing effect. They can offer temporary relief from the pain of aching muscles or that of a muscle spasm. Used at bedtime, they can ease pain enough to promote sleep.

In all but severe cases of fibromyalgia, the suppression of pain (barring that of flare-ups) can most safely be achieved by taking painkillers in lower quantities. Practicing self-help pain management, a gentle exercise program and improved posture can go a long way toward alleviating pain without these negative effects. It is important, too, to learn to read your body. Painkillers taken before the pain intensifies are far more effective than painkillers taken when the pain is already severe.

Narcotic analgesia

Prescription painkillers that combine acetaminophen and sometimes caffeine with codeine are tightly controlled in the U.S. Fears of addiction have long prevented doctors from prescribing narcotic medications to chronic pain patients. However, many experts now claim that this important form of analgesia has been mistakenly withheld. We all know how addictive heroin and cocaine are, how the user can rapidly become a "junkie." Codeine and morphine are fellow narcotics, yet when used carefully to suppress chronic pain their addictive qualities are debatable. This is because codeine and morphine are unlikely to hit the "pleasure zone" in the brain, and it is only when a drug hits the pleasure zone that the person craves more of the drug.

The fear of addiction was born after a 1998 study[6] into the effect of morphine on terminally ill cancer patients. When escalating doses were required to achieve the same level of pain relief, doctors wrongly concluded that the drug was becoming less efficient. We now know that, in fact, the cancers had actually spread, causing increased pain, which required increasing amounts of the medication.

This error aside, because the body is adept at adjusting to changes within itself, long-term use of narcotic medication can actually cause the body to set up additional pain receptors, and for this reason short-term use only is recommended. During attacks of acute pain, such as that experienced in a flare-up, narcotic medication can be very effective. It can not only relax a muscle spasm, it can also temporarily relieve anxiety and induce sleep—though not the deep sleep required in fibromyalgia—without fear of tolerance (where the patient needs to take escalating amounts to achieve the same effect). However, as with most medications, there are side effects. Narcotics can affect judgement, dexterity and short-term memory. They may even cause dizziness and nausea. All in all, when narcotics are treated with a lot of respect, they can be very useful.

Non-steroidal Anti-inflammatory Drugs (NSAIDs)

NSAIDs have both anesthetic and anti-inflammatory qualities. They can be used to control the aches and pains of many disorders, particularly the most common forms of arthritis. However, because fibromyalgia is not a true inflammatory disorder, NSAIDs are only useful in flare-ups. Dizziness and nausea can arise in the short term, while prolonged usage can cause stomach and bowel irritation. Taking NSAIDs with meals can reduce or eliminate side effects. As there are about a hundred medications in this category, your doctor may want to see how you respond to different ones. The only NSAID in tablet form available over the counter is Ibuprofen.

Over-the-counter anti-inflammatory gels are rarely strong enough to minimize the pain of a muscle spasm or flare-up. Prescription gels such as Feldene (piroxicam) massaged three times a day into painful areas, are known to be more useful, though.

Antidepressants

Antidepressants are frequently the first line of treatment for fibromyalgics—the primary objective being to boost serotonin levels. Fibromyalgia sufferers, as we have seen, have low supplies of this important chemical.

In treating fibromyalgia, antidepressants are usually prescribed in lower doses than when used solely to treat depression. Depression in fibromyalgia is now seen as a reaction to the condition, rather than a cause of it.

Tricyclic antidepressants

Medications belonging to the tricylic group of antidepressants are most successful in reducing the pain of fibromyalgia. They work by increasing the concentration of certain chemicals (one of them being serotonin) that are necessary for nerve transmission in the brain and spinal cord. These chemicals are known to promote sleep, reduce pain levels and ease muscle tension. To prevent the feeling of a "thick head" the following morning, tricyclic antidepressants are best taken in the evening rather than immediately before bedtime.

Tricyclic medications have several possible side effects. These include foggy brain, weight gain, constipation, dizziness, nausea, sweating, dry mouth and short-term memory problems. Taking this type of medication with food will lessen the chance of digestive problems.

There are many types of tricyclic antidepressants, all of which must be taken strictly as prescribed.

Muscle Relaxants

Muscle relaxants decrease muscle tension and are therefore useful for treating muscle spasms. They also help promote sleep. As long-term usage carries a high risk of tolerance and eventual dependency, it is not advisable to habitually use muscle relaxants to improve sleep. Also your doctor must be informed of any side effects, which may include dizziness, drowsiness, fatigue, flushing, headaches, nausea and nervousness.

When used to treat anxiety, medications in this category are very effective in the short term. It is important, however, to endeavor to discover the root cause of the problem—by seeing a trained counselor, for example. When used to treat muscle tension, muscle relaxants are recommended for pain flare-ups only—and then never for longer than four weeks at a time. Listen very carefully to your doctor's advice before taking this type of medication.

Trigger Point Injections

Usually lying at the center of fibrotic bands of muscle, trigger points are areas of acute sensitivity that, when "activated" (by overexertion, cold or a fall, for example), radiate pain into other areas. Anesthetic injections—which should be administered only by pain specialists familiar with the fibromyalgia condition—work by breaking the cycle of pain within the tissues. The actual location of the injection—that is, whether or not it hits the most troublesome spot—determines the level of pain relief. Dry needling can be enough to break the pain cycle, but most specialists prefer to inject anesthetic.

In most cases of fibromyalgia, the introduction of gentle exercise should then improve the quality of the tissues, gradually deactivating the trigger point and thereby reducing the radiated pain. The anesthetic Xylocaine (lidocaine) and its derivatives are most effective. It acts for an average of three weeks, but continued benefit depends on whether or not the patient can successfully improve muscle tone during that time.

Epidural Anesthetics

Where trigger point pain is severe and when anesthetic injections fail to improve the situation, some pain specialists may consider administering an epidural anesthetic. In this instance, anesthetic is injected into the epidural space within the spinal column. This space lies between the vertebral canal and the dura mater (outer membrane) of the spinal cord. It is important that the procedure be carried out under X-ray guidance.

In cases of acute inflammation—that is, where bursitis is apparent (bursitis is inflammation of the fluid in the hollow that protects and surrounds a joint)—or when inflammation has occurred around the spinal cord, the anesthetist may mix a steroidal medication with the anesthetic. Obviously a high degree of precision is required for this procedure and you should ensure that your anesthetist is well practiced in this field.

Pain levels generally decline for longer periods than they do after trigger point injections, giving the patient more time to improve the soft tissue situation.

Lidocaine Infusions

Lidocaine infusions generally involve a stay in the hospital. The patient has first to be assessed to ensure suitability for this type of pain relief. Blood tests and blood pressure readings are taken and the heart monitored by electrocardiogram (EKG). If all is well, the patient will be admitted about a week later.

During the first day in hospital, a fine tube (called a canula) is fitted and lidocaine anesthetic medication administered by drip. The patient is wired to a heart monitor and their blood pressure is measured regularly. The daily infusion can take six to eight hours to complete and is administered over several days.

As with trigger point injections and epidural anesthetics, this treatment allows the patient a little "breathing space" in which, with gentle exercise, the muscles can become stronger and more pliant.

4

Posture and Exercise

*I didn't know whether to laugh or cry when I was told that if I improved
my posture and exercised regularly my pain would gradually lessen!
Can't people understand that pain makes me slump and that exercise is
simply agonizing?*

Maintaining correct posture as we go about our daily activities is not
easy. It demands that we are constantly aware of how we carry ourselves and that we always seek the easiest way to perform tasks. Our
efforts in this area really are worth while, however, because repeated
stress on muscles affected by fibromyalgia can gradually cause pain
levels to rise.

Correct Posture

How often were we told, "sit up straight," "don't round your shoulders,"
"hold your head high" and "don't slouch" when we were young?
Slouching felt comfortable, though, and still feels easier than standing
or sitting erect.

Slouching may feel comfortable, but it stresses the muscles. After
years of slouching, healthy people may suffer occasional discomfort in
their lower backs, or they may experience an occasional twinge between
their shoulder blades. People with fibromyalgia don't get off so lightly.
Our reduced pain threshold means that poor posture can lead to
intensely troublesome pain.

Unfortunately, maintaining proper posture is a real problem for fibromyalgics. Keeping our backs straight, our heads held high under the burden of severe pain is awfully hard work. Pain drags us down; it makes us want to hang our heads; it makes our bodies want to sag. Sadly, though, poor posture has the effect of encouraging further pain, which in turn causes our posture to deteriorate further. It is another of those vicious circles that keep appearing in relation to fibromyalgia. Unless we learn to break out of these circles, our pain levels may continue to rise.

Breaking out of the vicious circle

Our backs consist of numerous internal and external muscles, all of which must be equally balanced in order to keep the lower back and pelvic regions correctly aligned. Activities that cause a shift in this alignment should be avoided—otherwise we risk incurring pain in our joints, muscles, ligaments and nerves.

Here are some basic postural recommendations that will help protect your body.

- When standing, make sure that your head sits over your shoulders and does not droop forward, and that your upper body is positioned directly over your feet (not with your hips forward so your spine forms an exaggerated "S" shape).
- Try at all times to retain the slight hollow in the middle region of your back. Whether you are still or performing an activity, your back should take on the form of an elongated "S" (not the exaggerated "S" mentioned above). Using a lumbar support will encourage the correct sitting posture.
- Stay relaxed. Maintaining correct posture does not mean tensing your muscles.
- Avoid slouching forward or leaning backward.
- Avoid twisting.
- Always have your work close to you.
- Warm up your muscles before performing any activity.
- Use the larger leg and arm muscles to perform tasks.
- Always seek the least physically stressful approach to an activity.
- Invest in energy-saving devices. Long-handled "grabbers" are quite useful, as are shopping carts on wheels, hands-free tele-

phones, electric can openers, electric carving knives and food processors.

- Be as mobile as possible. Maintaining one position for an extended period aggravates the muscles. Keep stretching and shifting position.
- Alternate work with rest periods.
- As soon as your pain levels begin to rise, stop what you are doing and consider your options. These may include getting help, taking a break or cancelling the activity altogether.

Advice for Specific Activities

Housework

That ceaseless task that needs doing in every home is a real source of frustration to people with fibromyalgia. You battle it at the expense of your health until finally you think you have it licked. Before you've recovered enough to sit back and appreciate your efforts, you realize it all needs doing again!

Before attempting housework of any kind, you should always consider the way you go about it. People with severe symptoms have little choice but to delegate most tasks to other family members. Encourage your children to earn their pocket money; explain to your partner that if they would take on the heavier work, they'll be rewarded by seeing you a lot less incapacitated. If your partner has no time for housework or if you live alone, paying a cleaner to do the necessary tasks may be an acceptable alternative.

However, it may be time to consider living in less than perfect conditions, at least for the duration of a difficult spell. Although kitchen hygiene should never be neglected, a little dust and disorder elsewhere can do no harm. Try to make pleasurable activities your first priority. Why make your symptoms worse doing housework just because you feel it is your duty or because you are worried that others will think badly of you for having a less than perfect home?

The following recommendations take into account both static and housework-oriented activities. Don't forget that before undertaking any activity you must assess whether or not you are physically up to it.

Try not to take chances, and don't be afraid to delegate. Asking for help does not signify weakness on your part. Asking for help takes guts. It is an essential part of coping with your fibromyalgia. Learning to accept assistance is a sure sign that you are coming to terms with your fibromyalgia. In accepting the illness, you make a giant leap toward dealing with it successfully.

Sitting for long periods

There are times when you may need to sit for long periods—waiting to see the doctor/dentist, watching a film or joining a family gathering, for example. Sitting can put a lot of stress on the back and hips.

- If possible, sit in a chair that supports your entire back. Chairs that look comfortable are not necessarily the most supportive. Your chosen chair should have adequate lumbar support and armrests and seat you higher than a standard armchair. The added height makes it easier for you to stand up. Orthopedic "high chairs" can be purchased from larger furniture retailers, as well as from specialist outlets. If you are not in your own home, choose the best chair available—if necessary, politely asking another person to vacate the best seat, briefly explaining why you need a supportive chair.
- Make sure you always adopt the correct sitting posture. Your bottom should be tucked well into the back of the seat, your spine supported by the back of the chair. Your head should sit directly on top of your shoulders so that your body carries its weight. Allowing your head to droop forward puts your neck muscles under terrific strain.
- Place a small cushion in the hollow of your back, around the level of your waist. This lumbar support encourages proper posture.
- Get up and walk around at regular intervals. If you are in someone else's home, explain that keeping as mobile as possible reduces your pain. If you are at the theater, say, try to purchase seats at the end of a row. That way you will not disturb people if you make regular trips to the restroom, bar, refreshment counter and so on to give your back a break. If you are waiting to see your doctor, dentist, rheumatologist or whomever, again,

get up and walk around as often as you can. Peruse the bulletin boards, take a couple of quick trips to the restroom, stand looking out of the window for a while. Don't worry about drawing attention to yourself; keeping your pain levels under control is of far more importance. If you are at home, remember not to sit for prolonged periods. When watching TV, use the commercial breaks to wander around—and "lose" the remote control. You may prefer to lay on the sofa awhile to give your back a break.

- If you are at home, place a hot water bottle on your back to relax the muscles. Requesting a hot water bottle from family and friends will help your back stand up to the strain of sitting when you are visiting their homes.

Leaning over to read or write

As your head is the approximate weight of a bowling ball—about 14 pounds—it exerts enormous strain on your neck muscles. Leaning with your head forward can severely stress your neck and upper/middle back. Such positioning can also cause headaches. It is best to do the following:

- Invest (or ask your employer to invest) in a chair that supports your whole back. If you are unable to find such a chair at regular furniture outlets, try a specialist.
- Move the chair as close to the desk or table as possible to encourage proper posture.
- Be sure you are sitting straight, with your bottom pressed to the back of the chair. This should prevent you leaning forward.
- Tuck in your chin as you look down to reduce neck strain.
- Bring your work closer to eye level. You may want to use a lap desk, drafting table or secure box placed on top of your usual desk or table.
- Place frequently used work materials within easy reach.
- Tilt your head back now and then to compensate for prolonged forward positioning.
- Take regular breaks. If you have a lot of paperwork to get through, keep getting up and walking around.
- Split the work into several short sessions. In the workplace, try to alternate "looking down" tasks with duties where you can be more mobile.

Typing

Using a computer or typewriter can stress the back, neck, shoulders, arms, wrists and hands. Here are some guidelines to minimize this:

- Follow the above recommendations for sitting at a desk or table.
- Use the computer's tilting feature to find the best position. When seated, the top line of the screen should be no higher than eye level. Positioning the screen too high will cause unnecessary neck strain.
- Make sure that the screen is directly opposite you. Looking to one side for prolonged periods can severely strain the neck muscles.
- If possible, adjust the height of your chair or work surface so your forearms are parallel with the floor and your wrists are straight. Sitting at a low work surface encourages poor posture.
- Invest in (or ask your employer for) a foot rest. This will reduce the pressure on your lower back.
- The mouse and other input devices should be positioned so that your arms and hands are in a relaxed and natural position.
- Position the keyboard directly in front of you. This makes it possible to type with your shoulders and arms relaxed.
- If you use a document holder, position it at the same level as the computer screen.
- Position the mouse at the same level as the keyboard.
- When typing, keep your wrists in a straight and natural position.
- Keep your elbows in a relaxed position by your sides.
- Use the minimum force required to push down the keys.
- Purchase an ergonomic wrist rest for your keyboard. This should help to reduce (or prevent) tendon pain—similar to that of repetitive motion injury—in your hands and wrists.
- Purchase (or ask your employer for) an ergonomic keyboard.
- Flex your hands and wrists every 10 minutes.
- If required, use a wrist splint to minimize wrist mobility.
- If using a conventional mouse, move it with your whole arm.
- If possible, use a computer mouse containing a trackball. This will limit wrist movement.
- Using an ergonomically "molded" mouse will support your hand and wrist.

- Take regular breaks. You will find that frequent, short breaks are far more beneficial than fewer, longer breaks.
- Stand and take a few minutes to stretch your muscles between breaks.
- Give yourself a time limit. When it is up, break off until later. (If your pain levels begin to rise before your time is up, finish what you are doing immediately.)

Reaching up to perform a task

Performing an activity while reaching upward—say, taking dishes down from a high shelf, replacing a light bulb, hanging curtains—can put your back, shoulders and arms under enormous strain. It is best to:

- stand on a small stool (one you know to be stable) so you don't have to stretch);
- use a long-handled implement for inaccessible cleaning jobs;
- take regular breaks to minimize strain;
- store items in general use—groceries, pans, dishes and so on— in more accessible cupboards.

Dishwashing, preparing vegetables and so on

Leaning over kitchen work surfaces for prolonged periods can stress the neck and back. It is best to:

- move as close to the work surface as possible to encourage proper posture;
- stand tall, making sure to tilt your head and tuck in your chin;
- place a wooden box on the work surface to bring the work closer (maybe you know a do-it-yourselfer who can make you one);
- take regular breaks;
- stop altogether as soon as you feel your normal pain levels begin to rise.

Carrying purchases and so on

Carrying heavy shopping bags and other items in your hands, arms extended, exerts great strain on your shoulders, arms and back. It is best to:

- park as close as possible to the supermarket or store;
- take someone with you so you can share the load;

- limit the amount you carry at one time—two trips carrying less is better than one trip carrying lots of bags or boxes;
- carry items close to your body, wrapping your arms around your packages; carrying loads close to the body disperses the strain;
- make sure the load is balanced;
- use a shopping cart on wheels, or ask a supermarket bagger to take your purchases to your car for you. You might also try using Internet or phone shopping services available in some cities that do the shopping and then deliver it to you.

Lifting a bulky object off the floor

Bending forward to lift something like a full laundry basket can strain the whole back—the lower back being particularly vulnerable. When lifting, you should be careful to ensure that your legs rather than your back take the strain. The golden rule is "LNB"—which stands for Legs Not Back. First of all you must assess whether or not you are really up to lifting. If you choose to go ahead, it is best to:

- plant your feet about 12 inches or so apart—a wide base helps maintain correct alignment;
- keeping your back straight, bend your knees until you are resting on your haunches, then place your arms around the object;
- push upward with your legs in order to raise it from the ground;
- if possible, break the load into smaller portions—where laundry is concerned, it is safer to lift a few items at a time, carrying them close to your body (perhaps over your arm if the items are dry) to the washing machine and drier; and
- if the object is larger than a laundry basket, get someone to help.

Carrying a bulky object

Because oxygen is not readily converted into energy in fibromyalgia, carrying can severely stress the hands, wrists, arms, shoulders, neck and back. It is best to:

- keep the object close to your body as you walk, making sure your grip on it is firm;
- maintain an upright posture, again ensuring that your legs—not your back—take the strain (LNB);

- rest the object on an available table or work surface to give your muscles a break during the carrying time.

Setting down a bulky object

Lowering a bulky object down on to the floor stresses the lower back in particular. It is best to:

- plant your feet about 12 inches apart;
- keeping your back straight, bend your knees, letting your legs take the strain as you lower the object to the floor;
- if transporting laundry from the kitchen to the outside clothes line, for example, setting the basket on a nearby patio table, garden bench or broad-topped wall will save you the strain of lowering it to the ground.

Picking something light up off the floor

Most people tend to arch right over to pick a piece of fluff, for example, off the carpet. This can put enormous strain on the back—the lower back in particular. It is best to:

- keep your back straight, bending your knees until you are able to reach the object;
- use your thigh muscles to propel you upright again;
- if your leg muscles are too weak or painful to do the above, use a long-handled "grabber."

Putting a casserole in an oven

Bending forward at the waist while carrying heavy things with your arms outstretched puts a great deal of stress on your back. Holding something heavy away from your body increases that strain. It also stresses the tissues of the hands, wrists, arms, shoulders and neck. If your oven is below worktop level, it is best to:

- stand close to the open oven, holding the casserole dish in both hands;
- drop down on to your haunches, keeping the dish close to your body, and slip the dish into the oven;
- push yourself upright again with your thigh muscles
- reverse the procedure to remove the casserole from the oven.

Putting laundry into the washing machine

Bending to push clothes into the washing machine can stress your back and shoulders. It is best to:

- lower yourself into a kneeling position, keeping your back straight;
- push only a small amount of washing in at a time—several repetitions are better than trying to thrust in a large bundle at once (reverse the procedure to remove the washing).

Lying in bed all night

Lying down for long periods can make you feel stiff and sore. In particular, lying on your back puts a lot of pressure on your back and hips. It is best to:

- place a pillow beneath your knees to take the strain off your lower back;
- use no more than one pillow to support your head and neck—molded cervical pillows keep the head correctly aligned during sleep;
- turn on to your side to relieve the pressure on your back and place a pillow between your knees to take the strain off your hips;
- don't sleep on your stomach;
- use a reasonably firm mattress—mattresses that sag will only aggravate your problems.

Driving a car

Driving can stress virtually every muscle in the body. It is important to assess whether or not you are up to driving in the first place. If you believe you are, it is best to:

- adjust the seat so it is near the steering column;
- make sure the back of the seat is adjusted correctly—it should be neither too upright nor reclined too far;
- don't slouch or allow your head to droop forward;
- wear an inflatable neck support;
- use a lumbar support (a cushion in the small of your back will suffice);

- make sure your car has a headrest and adjust it to suit your height—in the unlucky event of a collision, the headrest can minimize the severity of whiplash injury;
- when driving, armrests can reduce stress on the arms, shoulders and upper back; they can also help support the upper back when you travel as a passenger;
- use your side mirrors when backing up rather than turn around unnecessarily;
- when buying a car, go for power steering if possible. Perform plenty of slow maneuvers when you take a car for a test drive, then pick a car with light steering—some cars, even small ones, can be surprisingly heavy to handle at slow speeds;
- choose a car with an automatic transmission, eliminating the need to depress the clutch and work the gearshift;
- electric windows, side mirrors, sunroof and so on are easier to manage than their manually controlled counterparts;
- make regular breaks in a long journey to walk around and stretch your muscles;
- share the driving with someone else.

When traveling as a passenger, follow the relevant steps above to ensure that you are sitting properly to minimize the stresses on your body.

Rising from a chair

Jerking your upper body forward to get out of your seat can stress the muscles of your entire back. It is best to:

- move your bottom to the edge of the seat;
- place one foot as far backward as possible;
- use the armrests to help propel you upward, making sure you don't lean forward as you stand.

Getting out of bed

Twisting your body to get out of bed (or off the sofa) can put the back and hips under a lot of strain. It is best to:

- roll onto your side, bending your knees so they hang slightly over the edge of the bed;
- move your feet outward and over the edge of the bed;

- place the palm of your overhead arm on the bed at the level of your waist and, as you push your body upward, swing your legs down until they touch the floor—this should smoothly propel you into a sitting position.

Exercise

For years we have known that inadequate exercise can aggravate fibromyalgia. Surprisingly, it is now widely believed that it can also contribute to the onset of the condition. Many people who develop fibromyalgia following a physical trauma report that their activity levels were reduced significantly following the initial trauma, probably for reasons of self-protection. Now that we are aware of this factor, it is hoped that at some point in the future, doctors will be able to slow down or even prevent the illness. This would be done by monitoring physical trauma patients—particularly those suffering whiplash injuries—more thoroughly. Ensuring they are taught correct posture and that they follow a home exercise regime should, hopefully, be a part of their post-trauma treatment.

Adopting a physical exercise program has long been hailed as being beneficial for fibromyalgics. In conjunction with other treatment regimes—improved diet, antidepressant medication, self-talk and so on—the improvements can be profound. Think about and choose your forms of exercise with care, making sure you do not decide on something that will be difficult to keep up because, for example, a class takes place some distance away. Be flexible, too, as variety keeps it interesting and enjoyable. Ensure there is something you can do whether you are well or not feeling so good.

Why exercise?

The majority of fibromyalgics have made efforts to exercise but are put off further attempts by a subsequent rise in their pain levels. After all, the knowledge that physical activity will, in all probability, generate further pain is far from encouraging. Bad experiences of exercise can not only decrease motivation, they can also induce exercise phobias.

It is a sad fact that when we first start an exercise program, the pain is likely to increase temporarily. This occurs because our muscles are tight and out of condition. However, unfortunately, the only way to stretch and strengthen the muscles is to exercise them. Without exercise our bodies are liable to become increasingly painful—prolonged inactivity, ultimately, causing our muscles to waste. However, any activity or exercise producing more than a slight increase in pain should immediately be curtailed.

An Individually Tailored Regime

The severity of the symptoms related to fibromyalgia varies considerably from person to person. The pain and fatigue also affects people differently. It is advisable, therefore, that each person develop a personalized routine. This routine should depend largely on which activities you are most able to do without provoking more pain, as well as on those you enjoy the most.

As you read through the exercise possibilities—given below in order of progression—mark the ones you think you may be able to do. Remember that even if only warm-ups may be within your scope at the outset, you should be able to expand your routine as your muscles gain in flexibility and strength.

Take care not to overdo it

Unfortunately, there are still some people who believe fibromyalgics simply need to "push themselves" in order to improve their condition. (If only it was that simple. . . .) Your doctor or physical therapist may even believe that regular vigorous exercise is the only way to increase depleted levels of certain growth hormones, which are essential for the repair and regeneration of the tissues. However, recent research has found that exercise does not increase the production of growth hormones in fibromyalgia. In fact, vigorous exercise is known to cause microscopic tears in the muscle tissues (microtraumas). In healthy people such tears may promote slight stiffness, but sufferers of fibromyalgia—a disease of pain amplification—often experience the tears as severe pain.

Don't let anyone tell you that although your pain may feel severe, your muscles are not badly affected. We now have evidence that strongly indicates that prolonged muscle pain causes pain-transmitting chemicals to continue to build, which, in turn, causes pain levels to continue to rise. The higher the levels of pain, the more stress and tension are induced. Because of this, any activity should be undertaken with extreme care.

It makes sense, then, to say that in attempting to formulate an exercise routine, it is important that fibromyalgics refrain from pushing themselves beyond their known limits. Although a little added discomfort should be expected, it should not exceed the stage where you will not recover with rest during the remainder of the day and overnight.

After warming up, perform one or two of the easier stretching exercises. If your stiffness, fatigue and pain levels remain higher than normal the following day, either you did not allow sufficient resting time for your body to recover or your chosen exercise was, in fact, over-ambitious. Allow your body another two or three days to recover, then recommence your routine with a more basic exercise, and make sure you get enough rest afterwards. As you finish your exercise routine, you should feel as if you could have done more. Bear in mind that you may be able to achieve the dropped exercise when your muscles are stronger.

I recommend that for several days you think carefully about all the exercises described. You may perhaps want to rank the exercises, placing an asterisk beside those you think you can attempt, then two asterisks beside the easier of them, starting your routine with these. You may decide to aim to do 15 minutes of exercise a day, but, to be safe, you should spend only 2 or 3 minutes exercising at the outset. On the other hand, your objective may be to exercise for an hour. This is not advisable. It is far safer to break exercise sessions into two parts, completing a second session later in the day if you still feel up to it.

Activities/movements to avoid

A contracted muscle will shorten and appear larger—such as a contracted biceps muscle, which bulges when the elbow is bent. Working muscles—those being exercised—move by means of "concentric contraction." Like a working bicep muscle, they, too, shorten and may appear larger. "Eccentric" contraction occurs when a muscle is shortened but is being forced to lengthen. This happens when you are lifting something and stretching at the same time—for example, when reaching to place a heavy pan on a high shelf. The biceps muscle contracts because the pain is heavy, yet you have to extend your arm to reach the shelf. Forcing muscles to stretch while they work can cause small tears in the muscle tissues, which take time to heal and can be very painful.

Identifying and eliminating eccentric muscle movement is an important part of reducing the pain of fibromyalgia. It can be learned, as long as you try to focus on all that you do. Vacuuming is a typical example of eccentric movement. You contract your muscles to grip the handle of the vacuum cleaner, yet at the same time you push it back and forth. For the same reason, loading a dishwasher is hard on the muscles, as are putting dishes away, hanging out laundry, gardening, hammering, sawing and so on.

You may be surprised to learn that swimming is not recommended for fibromyalgics either. Although the water supports the body, the arm movements required for most strokes involve this eccentric contraction. Water exercises can be a beneficial alternative, however, and you may want to join an aqua-aerobics class

Warm-up Exercises

Many muscle groups are permanently tight and prone to being painful. If you try to move them beyond a certain point, they may resist, and forcing them only makes them more painful. It is essential, therefore, to perform warm-up exercises at the start of your routine. Warm-ups should include mobility exercises for your joints, simple pulse-raising activities for your heart and lungs and short, static stretches for your muscles.

Although I have described the warm-up exercises recommended for fibromyalgics generally, the ones you choose should depend on your own limitations. For example, a person with severe symptoms would be advised to formulate a very gentle program. One or two repetitions of several exercises are usually better than several repetitions of only one or two exercises. A person with milder symptoms can devise a more challenging program, lasting maybe 15 to 30 minutes. In the latter instance, warm-ups should last up to 10 minutes and be slightly more energetic.

Note: Never skip warm-ups in favor of more vigorous exercise.

Mobility exercises

These exercises should be smooth and continuous. It is important, too, that you keep your body relaxed. Exercising when tense can cause more harm than good. Remember to keep your back straight, your bottom tucked in and your stomach flattened as you perform your routine. You should stand with your legs slightly apart.

SHOULDERS

Letting your arms hang loose, slowly circle your shoulders backward. Repeat the exercise two to 10 times, depending on your condition. Now slowly circle your shoulders forward and repeat between 2 and 10 times, as appropriate.

NECK

1. Making sure you are standing straight, slowly turn your head to the left—as far as it will comfortably go—then hold for a count of two. Return to the center and repeat the exercise between 2 and 10 times. Now turn your head to the right, holding for a count of two before returning to center. Repeat between 2 and 10 times.

2. Tucking in your chin, tilt your head down and hold for a count of two. Repeat between 2 and 10 times. Again tucking in your chin, tilt your head upward, but not so far that it virtually sits on your shoulders, and hold for a count of two. Repeat between 2 and 10 times.

SPINE

1. Placing your hands on your hips to help support your lower back, slowly tilt your upper body to the left and hold for a count of two. Return to the center, then repeat between 2 and 10 times. Now tilt to the right and return to the center. Repeat between 2 and 10 times (*see Figure 3*).

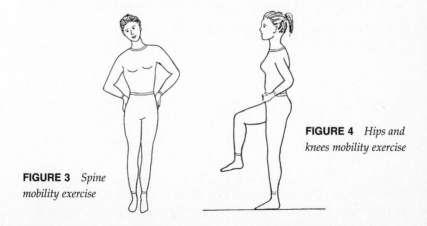

FIGURE 4 *Hips and knees mobility exercise*

FIGURE 3 *Spine mobility exercise*

2. Keeping your lower back static, gently, swing your arms and upper body to the left as far as it will comfortably go in a flowing rather than fast movement, then return to the center. Repeat between 2 and 10 times. Now swing your arms and upper body to the right and return to the center. Repeat between 2 and 10 times.

Hips and knees

With your body upright, move your hips by lifting your left knee upward, as far as is comfortable. Hold for a count of two, then lower. Now raise your right knee and hold for a count of two. Repeat between 2 and 10 times (*see Figure 4*).

Ankles

With your supporting leg slightly bent, place your left heel on the floor in front of you. Lift up your left foot and then place your left toes on the floor. Repeat between 2 and 10 times. Now duplicate the exercise and number of repetitions with the right foot (*see Figures 5A and 5B*).

Pulse-raising activities

Still part of your warm-up routine, pulse-raising activities must be gentle and should build up gradually. Their purpose is to help warm your muscles in preparation for stretching. Walking around the room for two to four minutes, followed by walking once up and down the stairs, is ideal.

Stretching exercises

The muscles, already becoming warm and flexible, relax further when short stretches follow mobility and pulse-raising activities. Stretches

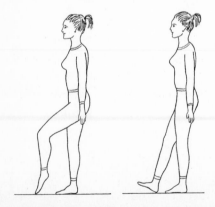

FIGURES 5A & 5B
Ankle mobility exercises

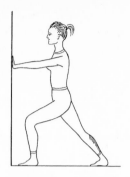

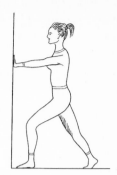

FIGURE 6 *Stretching exercise for the calves*

FIGURE 7 *Stretching exercise for the front of the thigh*

prepare them for the more challenging movements that follow. Again, it is up to you to decide which you think you are capable of performing. On days when you feel a little more delicate than usual, carrying out a few stretching exercises should help to relax the muscles.

CALVES

1. Stand with your arms outstretched, your palms against a wall. Keeping your left foot on the floor, bend your left knee and stretch your right leg out behind you. Press the heel of your right foot into the floor until you feel a gentle stretch in your leg muscles. Now switch legs. Repeat between 2 and 10 times (*see Figure 6*).

2. Standing with your feet slightly apart, raise both heels off the floor so that you are on your toes. Repeat between 2 and 10 times. As your calf muscles strengthen, you should be able to stay on your toes for longer periods of time. This exercise also helps your balance.

FRONT OF THE THIGHS

Using a chair or wall for support, stand with your left leg in front of your right, both knees bent, your right heel off the floor. Tuck in your bottom, and move your hips forward until you feel a gentle stretch in the front of your right thigh. Now change over legs. Repeat between 2 and 10 times (*see Figure 7*).

BACK OF THE THIGHS

Stand with your legs slightly bent, your left leg back about 8 inches in front of your right leg. Keeping your back straight, place both hands on your hips and lean forward a little. Now straighten your left leg, tilting

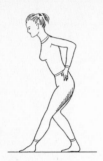

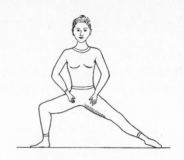

FIGURE 8 *Stretching exercise for the back of the thighs*

FIGURE 9 *Stretching exercise for the inner thigh*

your bottom back until you feel a gentle stretch in the back of your left thigh. Now change over legs. Repeat between 2 and 10 times (*see Figure 8*).

INNER THIGHS

Spreading your legs slightly, your hips facing forward and your back straight, bend your left leg, and keeping the right leg straight, move it slowly sideways until you feel a gentle stretch along your inner thigh. Gently move to the right, bending your right leg as you straighten the left (*see Figure 9*).

CHEST

Keeping your back straight, your knees slightly bent and your pelvis tucked under, place your arms as far behind your lower back as you can

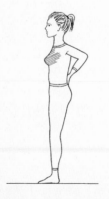

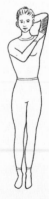

FIGURE 10 *Stretching exercise for the chest*

FIGURE 11 *Stretching exercise for the back of the upper arm*

and your hands gently on your lower back. Now move your shoulders and elbows back until you feel a gentle stretch in your chest (*see Figure 10*).

BACK OF THE UPPER ARMS

With your knees slightly bent, your back straight and your pelvis tucked under, raise your left arm and bend it so that your hand drops behind your neck and upper back. Using your right hand, apply slight pressure backward and downward on your left elbow, until you feel a gentle stretch (*see Figure 11*).

Note: Most fibromyalgics have some muscle groups that are far tighter than others—often the neck and shoulders. To reduce the gradual build-up of pain in these areas, you will benefit from gently stretching the relevant muscle groups at intervals throughout the day.

Strengthening Exercises

Not all fibromyalgics can tolerate strengthening exercises, so use caution, beginning with one or two repetitions of your chosen exercises. Although the movements may seem easy at the time, the real test is how you feel the next morning.

The following exercises help condition the muscles required for pushing, pulling and lifting. They will also increase your stamina. Remember to incorporate small pauses between repetitions, focus on staying relaxed and don't forget to breathe as you exercise.

THIGHS

1. The large muscles running along the tops of your thighs (the quadriceps) quickly become weak when you are inactive. Strengthening exercises will help you walk, climb stairs and get in to and out of chairs more easily. Lean back against a wall, your feet a foot away from the base of the wall. Adopting correct posture, slowly squat down, keeping your heels on the ground. (Don't go too far down at first.) Now slowly straighten your legs again. Repeat between 2 and 10 times, lowering yourself farther as, over time, your muscles strengthen.

2. Holding onto a sturdy chair and keeping your back "tall," bend and then slowly straighten both legs keeping your heels on the floor. Repeat the exercise between 2 and 10 times (*see Figure 12*).

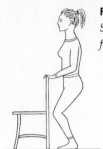

FIGURE 12
*Strengthening exercise
for the thighs*

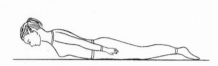

FIGURE 13 *Strengthening exercise
for the upper back*

3. Sit in a chair and push your knees together, tightening your muscles as you do so. Hold for a few seconds. Repeat between 2 and 10 times.

UPPER BACK

Lie face down on the floor, hands by your side, not on the floor, and keeping your legs straight and tightening your stomach and back muscles, gently raise your head and shoulders. Hold for a count of two, then lower. Repeat between 2 and 10 times (*see Figure 13*).

LOWER BACK

Lie on your back, using a small rolled cloth or towel to support your neck, then lift your knees, keeping your feet on the floor. First lift your left leg gently behind the knee, pulling it towards your chest until you feel a gentle pull in your bottom and lower back. Repeat with the right leg. Now pull both legs up together. Repeat each exercise between 2 and 10 times (*see Figure 14*).

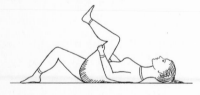
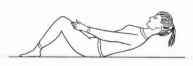

FIGURE 14 *Strengthening exercise
for the lower back*

FIGURE 15 *Strengthening exercise
for the abdomen*

ABDOMEN

1. The abdominal muscles commonly become very weak in people with fibromyalgia. However, the stronger they are, the more they support your back. Lie on your back, using a small rolled cloth or towel to support your neck. Lift your knees and place your feet flat on the floor. Now tighten your abdominal muscles, tuck your chin in a little towards your chest and raise your head and shoulders, reaching your arms toward your knees. Remember to keep your lower back pressed down on the floor (*see Figure 15*).

2. If you are not doing sit-ups, the following exercise is just as effective. Lie on your back, using a small rolled cloth or towel to support your neck. Pull in your stomach muscles and try to flatten your spine against the floor. Hold for a count of two, then release. Repeat 2 to 10 times

ARMS

Place your left hand on your chest and press for a few seconds. Do the same with your right arm. Repeat between 2 and 10 times.

PUSH-UPS

Stand up with your hands flat against a wall, your body straight. Carefully lower your body towards the wall, then slowly push away. Repeat 2 to 10 times. At first, stand quite near the wall, then try moving farther away as you become stronger (*see Figures 16A and 16B*).

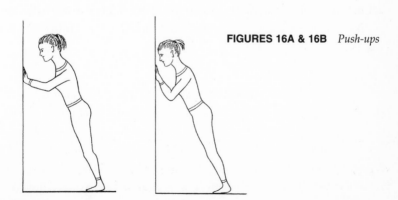

FIGURES 16A & 16B   *Push-ups*

USING SMALL WEIGHTS

People with milder symptoms may now be able to increase their strength by using small weights. The type that fasten with Velcro around the wrists and ankles are recommended. Weights of 8 ounces each slip into small pockets sewn into the band. Such weights are available from most sports shops. Start by using one weight only.

1. With the weights around your wrists, stand with your feet slightly apart. Making sure that only your upper body moves, turn carefully to the left, swinging both arms gently as you move. Repeat two or three times. Now perform the same exercise and number of repetitions, but this time swing your body and arms to the right. Be sure the movements are steady and fluid, not too fast.

2. Keeping your left elbow close to your waist, slowly raise your left forearm so it almost touches your shoulder. Lower the forearm until it is at right angles with your upper arm, then slowly raise it again. Now repeat the exercise with your right arm, again ensuring your movements are steady and continuous.

3. Bending your left arm, bringing your hand up until your wrist is level with your shoulder, reach your hand upwards until your wrist is level with your shoulder. Bring it straight back down to the original position. Repeat once more, then do the same with your right arm.

As you gain in strength and flexibility you may, first of all, be able to increase the number of repetitions you do and, second, to add to the weight you lift. If your pain levels are higher than normal the next day, however, I recommend that you postpone these exercises until you feel stronger.

WALKING WITH WEIGHTS

Using the Velcro weight bands described above as you walk around the house, up and down the stairs or on a treadmill can strengthen your leg, hip and back muscles and help to protect against osteoarthritis. Strap the weight bands to your ankles, placing one weight in each. Walk a few steps to determine your response. If later, you only feel slight discomfort, repeat the exercise everyday until the discomfort dissipates. Next, increase the time spent wearing the weight bands, then slowly add more weights. Note, however, that some people may not be able to tolerate this exercise at all.

GRIPPERS

Squeezing cushioned "hand-grippers" between your thumbs and fingers can greatly increase the strength and dexterity of your hands. Furthermore, almost all fibromyalgics will be able to perform this exercise, slowly and steadily increasing the number of repetitions. Hand-grippers can be purchased at most sports shops.

Aerobic Exercise

Because the muscle fibers in fibromyalgics are unable to adequately utilize oxygen, aerobic exercise is beneficial. It actually has been proven to significantly reduce the pain and fatigue of the condition. The improvements may be due to the fact that aerobic exercise releases "feel-good" endorphins—the "natural" painkillers. In addition, muscle temperature rises, helping them to relax, so they receive more oxygen and waste products are removed more efficiently. The cardiovascular system also benefits from aerobic exercise, helping to protect against heart disease and improving circulation. Regular aerobic activity also carries the added bonuses of increasing your stamina levels and helping you lose weight.

The strengthening exercises described above should be performed for at least two weeks before embarking on aerobic activity. The increased muscle capacity that results from doing the strength training allows greater benefit to be gained from aerobic activity.

Ideally, you should then aim to develop a program involving a small amount of aerobic activity, preferably of the low-intensity type. Jogging on a hard floor or road, using a rowing machine or any multi-gym equipment is not recommended for fibromyalgics.

Note: Check with your doctor before going ahead with any aerobic activity.

Types of low-impact aerobic activities

The following activities are listed in order of difficulty. If you feel able to perform more than one, be sure to work through them in the order given.

WALKING

Always be sure you choose an aerobic exercise you enjoy and one that is within your physical and practical scope. Walking is good. It is a weight-bearing activity that increases mobility, strength, stamina and helps protect against osteoporosis. If your symptoms are severe, you may just want to walk to the nearest lamppost and back on your first day. On the second and third days, you should try and repeat that. On the fourth day, you could try walking to the second lamppost, on the fifth and sixth days to repeat that, on the seventh day to the third lamppost, on the ninth and tenth to repeat that and so on. For most people, walking is the easiest and most convenient aerobic activity. You may surprise yourself at how far you can actually walk, after increasing the distance over several weeks.

However, you must be weary of walking outdoors in cold, damp conditions. An electrically operated treadmill can, if you can afford the initial outlay, be an excellent investment. It will give you the freedom to walk for as long as you want in the winter as well as summer, whatever the weather. Also, a treadmill offers a continuous level walking, people with lower back, hip and leg pain may walk far greater distances this way than they could hope to over the variable terrain found outdoors. Although some people consider treadmill walking too monotonous and artificial, this can, to some extent, be overcome by reading a book or a magazine at the same time. Wearing a Walkman so you can listen to your favorite music, the radio or to stories and books on tape passes the time quickly, too. However, this said, treadmills should never wholly replace outdoor walking. Fresh air and sunlight are also important factors in lessening the effects of fibromyalgia.

STEPPING

Although greatly beneficial, not everyone with fibromyalgia will be able to perform step exercises. If you think you may be able to manage, you should start with a small step, such as a wide hefty book, or maybe a catalog or telephone directory. Make sure it is placed securely against a bottom stair to keep it steady and so that you have room to move (After two or three weeks, you may be able to use the bottom stair itself.) Place your left foot, the your right foot on the book or step. Now step backwards with first your left foot, then your right foot. Repeat between 2 and 10 times, then alternate your feet, placing first your right foot, then your left. You may eventually be able to perform the exercise for five or ten minutes.

TRAMPOLINE JOGGING

Jogging on a small circular trampoline can, if care is taken, be good aerobic exercise. Become accustomed to the feel of it by, at first, simply lifting your heels—not your feet—as if you were walking. If you can manage to get into a rhythm, the trampoline will do much of the work for you. Continue for two to three minutes.

Walking on the spot should be your next aim and then gentle jogging a while after that, if you can. Don't get carried away, though! Sharp jolts and jerks may do more harm than good. Small, inexpensive trampolines are available from most sports shops.

AQUA–AEROBICS

Although swimming can be counter-productive for fibromyalgics, aqua-aerobics, sometimes called "aqua-cizes," can be a pleasing and beneficial alternative. Because the water supports your body as you exercise—when you are submerged to the neck, you bear only about a tenth of your body weight—it moves the shock factor, conditioning your muscles with the minimum of discomfort. The pressure of the water also causes the chest to expand, encouraging deep breathing and increased oxygen uptake.

Rather then exercising alone in the pool, most people prefer to join aqua-aerobics classes. As well as providing encouragement and ensuring that you exercise properly for maximum benefit, this can bring you into contact with sufferers of similar health problems, such as arthritis, so you can empathize with, and support, each other. Most public swimming pools run aqua-aerobics sessions, some which are graded according to ability. You should inform the instructor of your limitations and avoid the more taxing exercises. I would advise that you phone, first of all, to check the water temperature since exercising in water below 84°F will cause your muscles to tighten—it may even induce a flare-up.

Aqua-aerobics, as with all types of exercises, is only truly beneficial when performed regularly. If you live a long way from a swimming pool, you will probably find yourself attending less and less as time goes by, then feel angry with yourself for giving up. To minimize feelings of failure, be wary of undertaking activities that it will be hard for you to keep doing regularly.

CYCLING

Whether using an exercise bike or an actual bicycle, this activity provides an efficient cardiovascular workout. However, caution must rule. People who suffer from lower back and buttock pain may, despite using a seat cushion, find that cycling aggravates the problem. Often the handlebars are too far forward, which can heighten neck, shoulder and upper back pain. Also, due to the continuous motion, your legs have no opportunity to rest, as they would between spells of most other types of exercise. Cycling, can therefore, create much pain for later.

It is best to start by pedaling slowly, gradually building momentum and, at first, limit your sessions to two or three minutes. After a month or so, people with milder symptoms may be able to cycle for 20 to 30 minutes. If you use an exercise bike, always set it at a low resistance level.

Cooling-down Exercises

Cooling down your muscles after exercise is just as important as warming them up beforehand. The longer stretches described below should only be done when your muscles are sufficiently warm, after exercise. Again, you should choose the exercises with which you know you can cope. If all the following are beyond your scope, repeat your choice of warm-up exercises instead. The cool-down phase should last up to five minutes.

CALVES

Keeping your right leg and back straight, place your palms against a wall, then bend your left knee (so that it extends farther than your left ankle). Press the heel of your right foot into the floor until you feel a gentle stretch. (Move your right foot farther back if yo don't feel a stretch.) Now exercise the other calf in the same way.

UPPER BACK

Sitting on the floor, your knees bent, hold on to your ankles and slowly round out your back. Pull in your stomach and lower your head until you feel a gentle stretch in the middle and upper parts of your back.

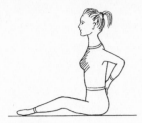

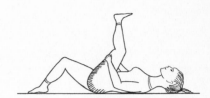

FIGURE 18   *Cooling-down stretch for the back of the thigh*

FIGURE 17   *Cooling-down stretch for the chest*

CHEST

Sitting on the floor, place your hands on your lower back, then move your shoulders back until you feel a gentle stretch in your chest (*see Figure 17*).

BACK OF THE THIGHS

Lie on your back, using a small rolled cloth or towel to support your neck, and lift both knees, keeping your feet flat on the floor. Now raise your left leg. Placing one hand behind and above your knee and the other behind and below it, slowly ease the leg toward your shoulders until you feel a gentle stretch along the back of your left thigh. Next, do the same with the right leg (*see Figure 18*).

FRONT OF THE THIGHS

Lying on your stomach, bend your left leg and hold your ankle with your nearest hand. Now, keeping your back straight, push your pelvis into the floor until you feel a gentle stretch along the front of your left thigh. Now do the same with the right leg (*see Figure 19*).

ABDOMINAL MUSCLES

Lying on your stomach, place your hands and forearms on the floor and slowly raise your upper body until you feel a gentle stretch in your abdominal muscles (*see Figure 20*).

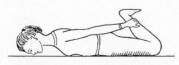

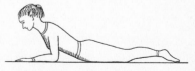

FIGURE 19   *Cooling-down stretch for the front of the thigh*

FIGURE 20   *Cooling-down stretch for the abdominal muscles*

Other exercises

The exercises "Back of the upper arms" (*Figure 11, page 56*) and "Thighs" (*Figures 7, 8 and 9, pages 55, 56*) should also be included in your cooling-down routine.

Getting Started on Your Routine

Have you checked with your doctor and made your choices? Have you selected the easier exercises with which you wish to start your routine? If so, you should now read the following recommendations. They should help to get you started with the minimum of discomfort.

First of all, it is advisable to exercise before your pain levels start to rise. It is important, too, that you set aside sufficient time to perform your routine—don't be tempted to rush.

- Relax your muscles by taking a warm shower shortly after waking.
- Eat a light breakfast to boost your energy levels—you should not exercise after a heavy meal.
- Dress in loose, comfortable clothing and good, supportive trainers.
- Be sure to exercise in a warm place, out of drafts.
- Start slowly and carefully. Only perform two or three repetitions of your chosen exercises. People with milder symptoms will be able to build up to 10 repetitions sooner than people with severe symptoms.
- Movements should be kept within your range. If you know that raising your arms past a certain level gives rise to pain in your shoulder, make sure you don't initially pass that level. You should actually be able to extend your range with time.
- As you exercise, keep checking your posture. When you allow your head and shoulders to droop, your back to slouch, you put added strain on your muscles. They then burn more energy, causing additional pain and fatigue.
- Take care that you don't involuntarily hold your breath when exercising. Breathe deeply and evenly, exhaling on the effort.

- Try to visualize the muscle group being exercised. This should prevent other muscle groups accidentally being worked.
- Pause between repetitions. There is a slight delay between muscle contraction and relaxation, so contracting a muscle without pausing means you do so when the muscle has already contracted. This causes a buildup of lactic acid in the area concerned, which, in turn, causes more pain.
- After exercising, it is important to allow time for recovery before attempting further activity. Don't berate yourself if your pain levels are surprisingly high afterwards. Get some extra rest, then begin a toned-down version of your routine as soon as you are able.
- When you finish you should feel as if you could have done more. This should help make sure you don't set yourself up for more pain for later.
- Don't try to make up for the days when you weren't able to do much. Set your limit at the start of each session and stick to it.

5

5

Complementary Therapies

*I was taking the appropriate medications, my eating habits had
improved and I was starting to exercise . . . I certainly felt better
physically, but I still needed extra help . . .*

Complementary medicine has been described as all the therapies not
taught in medical school. These include acupuncture, aromatherapy,
chiropractic, homeopathy, osteopathy and reflexology, among others.
You may know these techniques as "alternative therapies," but this
term for them can be misleading. The word "alternative" suggests that
it can be used to replace conventional medicine. Unfortunately, for
chronic pain conditions, this is rarely the case.

Complementary therapies are suitable for chronic pain sufferers
for the following reasons:

- they are relatively non-invasive;
- they are largely free from side effects;
- they can be used in addition to long-term medication;
- most of them are enjoyable—the "patient" can often relax completely, especially during the touch and massage techniques.

In a survey I carried out in 1998 on the members of the support
group in my area, the most popular complementary therapy was aromatherapy, closely followed by reflexology, acupuncture and chiropractic. It seemed that no one had tried homeopathy, acupressure, the
Bowen technique, Bach Flower Remedies or bioelectromagnetic thera-

py. However, I know that, following an introductory speech by a registered homeopathic practitioner and after the questionnaires were completed and returned, several members, including myself, are now finding homeopathic remedies very helpful. I believe that most of the other therapies were not tried simply because they were not readily available.

People who use complementary therapies do report substantial benefits, although some of this may be the result of knowing that they are doing something positive to help themselves. Different techniques seem to suit different people, so try some and see what works best for you.

Aromatherapy

Aromatherapy uses our sense of smell in the treatment of certain health disorders. Concentrated aromatic, or essential, oils are extracted from plants and may be inhaled, mixed with a carrier oil and rubbed directly into the skin, or used in bathing. Each scent relates to its plant of origin, so lavender oil has the same scent as the lavender plant and geranium smells like the geranium plant.

Plant essences have been used for healing throughout the ages, smaller amounts being used for aromatherapy purposes than for herbal medicines. The highly concentrated aromatherapy oils are obtained either by steaming a particular plant extract until the oil glands burst or by soaking the plant extract in hot oil so that the cells collapse and release their essence.

Techniques used in aromatherapy

INHALATION

Effecting the quickest result, inhalation of essential oils has a direct influence on the olfactory (nasal) organs and these are immediately received by the brain. Steam inhalation is the most popular technique. This can be achieved either by mixing a few drops of oil with a bowlful of boiling water or by using an oil burner whereby a candle heats a small container of water to which a few drops of oil have been added.

MASSAGE

Essential oils intended for massage are diluted before use. They should never be applied directly to the skin in an undiluted (pure) form. When using undiluted essential oils, mix three or four drops with a neutral carrier oil, such as olive or safflower oil. The oils penetrate the skin and are absorbed by the body, exerting a positive influence on a particular organ or set of tissues.

BATHING

Tension and anxiety can be reduced by using certain aromatherapy oils in the bath. A few drops of one or more pure essential oils should be added directly to running tap water. It mixes more efficiently this way than if it is added after you have turned off the taps. No more than 20 drops of oil in total should be added to bathwater.

Lavender is the most popular oil for use in the bath. It is a wonderful restorative and excellent for relieving tension headaches as well as stress.

Ylang-ylang has relaxing properties. It has a calming effect on the heart rate and can be used to relieve palpitations and raised blood pressure.

Chamomile can be very soothing. It aids both sleep and digestion, as well as being a good pain reliever.

As aromatherapy is a holistic therapy (where the practitioner looks at the person and their ills as part of the whole), questions about lifestyle, family circumstances and so on will be asked. Depending on your answers, a suitable essential oil or oils will be recommended. Many qualified aromatherapists offer a massage using the chosen oil(s). As well as being beneficial healthwise, aromatherapy massages are very relaxing.

If you are unable to consult with a qualified aromatherapist, your local health food store may provide you with details about which essential oils are appropriate for your needs. Alternatively, you may want to borrow a good aromatherapy book from the library.

Acupressure

Acupressure is an ancient form of oriental healing, combining acupuncture and massage. Practitioners of this technique use the thumbs, fingertips or palms of the hands to firmly massage certain pressure points, located at specific sites throughout the body. These points are the same as those used in acupuncture. Neither oils nor equipment are used in this type of therapy.

Acupressure is believed to enhance the body's own healing mechanisms. Pain relief is sometimes rapid. However, improvements can take longer in chronic pain conditions. At some hospitals, acupressure is available as part of the physical therapy treatment

Acupuncture

Also an ancient form of oriental healing, acupuncture involves puncturing the skin with fine needles at specific points of the body. These points are located along energy channels (meridians) which are believed to correspond with certain internal organs. This energy is known as *chi*. Emotional, physical or environmental factors are believed to disturb the *chi* energy balance. Needles are inserted to increase, decrease or unblock the flow of *chi* energy so that the balance of yin and yang is restored. Yin, the female force, is calm and passive; it also represents dark, cold, swelling and moisture. On the other hand, yang, the male force, is stimulating and aggressive, representing heat, light, contraction and dryness. It is thought that an imbalance of these forces is the cause of illness and disease. For example, a person who feels the cold and suffers fluid retention and fatigue would be considered to have an excess of yin. A person suffering from headaches, however, will be deemed to have an excess of yang.

Acupuncture is now losing its unorthodox reputation, and is generally accepted in the Western world. For example, acupuncture is used to alleviate stress, digestive disorders, insomnia, asthma and allergy. It is also documented as being successful in relieving pain.

A qualified acupuncturist will use a set method to determine which acupuncture points to use—it is thought there are as many as 2000 acupuncture points on the body. At a consultation, questions will be asked about lifestyle, sleeping patterns, fears, phobias and reactions to stress. The pulses will be felt, then the acupuncture itself carried out. The first consultation will normally last an hour, and patients should feel improvement after four to six sessions.

Bach Flower Remedies

In the 1930s, the philosophy of a Harley Street doctor, Edward Bach (pronounced "batch"), was "a healthy mind ensures a healthy body."

He was a man far ahead of his time, considering that mind and body are only now being more widely seen as closely linked.

Dr. Bach devised a method of treating the negative emotional state behind any disorder. First he sectioned emotional states into seven major groups—such as fear, loneliness, uncertainty—then he categorized 38 negative states of mind under each group. Using his knowledge of homeopathy, he went on to formulate a plant- or flower-based remedy to treat each of these emotional states, as follows:

1. *Fear*
   - For terror, he formulated Rock Rose remedy.
   - For fear of known things, he formulated Mimulus.
   - For fear of mental collapse, he formulated Cherry Plum.
   - For fears and worries of unknown origin, he formulated Aspen.
   - For fear or overconcern for others, he formulated Red Chestnut.

2. *Loneliness*
   - For impatience, he formulated Impatiens.
   - For self-centeredness/self-concern, he formulated Heather.
   - For pride and aloofness, he formulated Water Violet.

3. *Insufficient interest in present circumstances*
   - For apathy, he formulated Wild Rose.
   - For lack of energy, he formulated Olive.
   - For unwanted thoughts or mental arguments, he formulated White Chestnut.
   - For lack of interest in the present, he formulated Clematis.
   - For deep gloom with no known origin, he formulated Mustard.
   - For failure to learn from past mistakes, he formulated Chestnut Bud.

4. *Despondency or despair*
   - For extreme mental anguish, he formulated Sweet Chestnut.
   - For self-hatred/sense of uncleanliness, he formulated Crab Apple.
   - For overresponsibility, he formulated Elm.
   - For lack of confidence, he formulated Larch.
   - For self-reproach or guilt, he formulated Pine.
   - For after-effects of shock, he formulated Star of Bethlehem.

- For resentment, he formulated Willow.
- For exhausted but struggling on, he formulated Oak.

5. *Uncertainty*
   - For hopelessness and despair, he formulated Gorse.
   - For despondency, he formulated Gentian.
   - For indecision, he formulated Scleranthus.
   - For uncertainty as to the correct path in life, he formulated Wild Oat.
   - For the seeker of advice and confirmation from others, he formulated Cerato.
   - For "Monday morning" feeling, he formulated Hornbeam.

6. *Oversensitivity to influences and ideas*
   - For weak will and subserviency, he formulated Centaury.
   - For mental torment behind a brave face, he formulated Agrimony.
   - For hatred, envy or jealousy, he formulated Holly.
   - For protection from change and outside influences, he formulated Walnut.

7. *Overcareful of the welfare of others*
   - For intolerance, he formulated Beech.
   - For overenthusiasm, he formulated Vervain.
   - For self-repression/self-denial, he formulated Rock Water.
   - For the selfishly possessive, he formulated Chicory.

In addition, the Rescue Remedy is appropriate to many everyday situations in which emotional upheaval occurs. It is made from a combination of five Bach flower remedies—Rock Rose, Clematis, Cherry Plum, Impatiens and Star of Bethlehem.

Bioelectromagnetics

Bioelectromagnetics is the study of how living organisms—all of which produce electrical currents—interact with magnetic fields. The electrical currents within our bodies are capable of creating magnetic fields that extend outside our bodies, and these fields can be influenced by external magnetic forces. In fact, specific external magnetism can actually produce physical and behavioral changes. Just as drugs induce a response in their target tissues, so low magnetic fields can produce a chosen biological response, but without the side effects associated with drugs. However, external magnetism should not be used by anyone who has a heart pacemaker.

External magnetism can not only correct abnormalities in the energy fields of patients with disease, effectively working as a healer, it is also capable of stabilizing a chronic condition, although not in every case. As a pain reliever, external magnetism has long been used in the Far East and is becoming ever more widely used, and much experimentation is currently taking place. Electromagnetic machinery creates a pulsed magnetic field that is used to aid the recovery of bone fractures, tendon and ligament tears, muscle injuries and so on. A small, light, comparatively inexpensive version can be purchased for easy-to-wear home use.

When placed directly over the site of aches, pains or injuries, external magnetism is called magnotherapy. The following are examples of magnotherapy products now on the market:

- *Seating*   Chairs containing magnets at specific sites are now available. They can help to relax tension and reduce or prevent stiffness arising from prolonged sitting.
- *Massage tools*   Claimed to be the fastest-working massage implement, a magnetic massager delivers stimulating vibration that can boost circulation and relax the muscles. The massager can easily be used on painful areas. The magnetic head is battery powered.
- *Mattress pads*   Available for one person in a double bed, a magnetic mattress is durable and light enough to take on vacation. Thicker, super-magnetized mattress pads are also available.
- *Pillow pads*   Usable as a pillow in bed, as well as for sitting, these pads are light and portable.

Also available are magnetized body, arm/leg, neck, elbow, wrist/carpal, thumb, back, knee and ankle wraps.

External magnetism in the form of a specially designed wrist appliance, worn like a wrist watch, is also believed to be effective in treating aches, pains and injuries in any region of the body. As with the other types of external magnetism, this appliance is said to improve the ability of the blood to carry oxygen and nutrients around the body. It is also believed to speed the removal of toxins and other waste products.

The Bowen Technique

This dynamic system of muscle and connective tissue therapy is revolutionizing pain management and other healthcare practices worldwide. Australian Tom Bowen, who pioneered the technique in the 1950s, had successfully treated approximately 13,000 patients annually—with 80 to 90 percent of them responding favorably after only one or two treatments—before the technique was documented and introduced into other countries. Now widely recognized as a safe and effective therapy, the practitioner performs a sequence of small, precise movements at specific points on the body. This provokes a stimulus that releases the tissues in the problem area(s), which, in turn, triggers the body's own healing mechanisms.

The therapy can be performed through light clothing, while the patient is in a reclined position. A session will normally take 30 to 45 minutes, including short breaks to allow the body time to adjust to each part of the treatment. The patient is then asked to drink a quart of water within the following few hours to aid the removal of toxins from the lymphatic system.

Patients normally find the treatment relaxing, and many report almost immediate improvements. Others may feel improvements over the following two or three weeks, as the first treatment takes full effect. Long-standing pain may be eliminated in some conditions after three to six weeks of treatment. In fibromyalgia, the pain can be notably reduced for substantial periods. Sufferers with mild symptoms may even reporting a total elimination of pain.

Chiropractic

Chiropractic is a non-invasive therapy used to alleviate pain by muscle manipulation and spinal adjustment. Muscles are held together and connected to the joints by myofascia—a tubelike lining encasing the muscles and attaching them to the bones. The elevated muscle tension prevalent in fibromyalgia may, at times of physical or emotional stress, cause the myofascia to bunch up, impeding the flow of oxygen to the muscle cells. The muscles shorten, straining the myofascia and tendinous attachments, limiting their movement and making them susceptible to tearing.

Microscopic tears in the muscle fibers are thought to intensify pain and muscle fatigue. This may, in part, also be due to the fact that adjoining muscles are unable to slide over them as easily as they should. Painful trigger points may develop where muscle and bone connect. This circumstance may even pull joints out of position so that they become fixated, which means that the joint will not return to its natural position by itself and is therefore more painful. Chiropractors specializing in soft tissue manipulation (or myofascial pain syndrome techniques) may be helpful in reducing trigger point and tender point pain and correcting bone misalignments and fixations.

At the initial consultation, a chiropractor will need to thoroughly evaluate your condition. This is normally done with the help of X-rays. Many chiropractors also use the following to treat patients.

- *Ultrasound machines* An ultrasound machine performs a micro-massage of the muscle by producing sound waves that penetrate the tissues. The round applicator is simply moved over the surface of a painful area to help reduce muscle tension and pain. Physiotherapists also use ultrasound.

- *Microcurrent stimulation* This may be used to duplicate the body's own healing frequencies. The stimulator produces a low-voltage microelectrical current that feels like non-painful tingling. This technique should help relax muscles, restore normal circulation to the region and reduce pain. It is considered excellent for reducing jaw pain.

- *Spinal adjustment by hand* This is another chiropractic technique, but one with which fibromyalgics may not be able to cope. A spring-loaded activator—a six-inch long device—may be used instead. The chiropractor will set a tension level to deliver a specific force. The tension should be low for fibromyalgics.

- *Massage* This may also be performed by a chiropractor. However, the chiropractor should take care to be gentle and not aggravate muscles that are already sore.

Finding the right chiropractor

I advise you to ask a chiropractor several important questions before deciding to schedule your first session. The nature of the treatment is such that the chiropractor needs to know about fibromyalgia if they are to help rather than hurt you.

"Do you understand what fibromyalgia is?" If the answer is "Yes," ask a few basic questions about the condition.

- "Are you aware that spinal adjustment can hurt fibromyalgics?" If the answer is "Yes," ask how this problem can be avoided.
- "Do you use X-rays in your initial assessment?"
- "What methods do you use—ultrasound, microcurrent stimulation and others?"
- "Do you offer help in devising an exercise program?"

It is imperative that the chiropractor you choose answers each of the above questions to your satisfaction. At your first consultation, be sure the chiropractor understands your full medical history—many fibromyalgics have a lengthy medical background. Remind your chiropractor to be gentle and be sure to speak up when a particular treatment hurts.

Herbal Remedies

Traditional Chinese herbal remedies have been used to great effect since antiquity and are still the most widely used medicines in the world. Thirty percent of modern medicines are made from plant-derived substances. However, because modern medicines frequently have side effects, herbal medicines are preferred by many people. Although natural, herbal remedies should still be used with caution. They can interact with orthodox medication, so inform your doctor before starting treatment. Indeed, many medical professionals are of the opinion that herbal medicines should not be taken without the advice of a trained herbal doctor.

Your chosen herbalist will check your pulse rate and the color of your tongue for clues as to which bodily organs are depleted of energy. The doctor will then write a prescription for very precise doses according to your needs. Tablets made from compressed herbal extracts are often given, but sometimes you will be given a bag of carefully weighed and ground dried roots, flowers, bark and so on. In the latter case, an "infusion" should be made by pouring boiled water directly on to the herbal mixture. It should be left to stand for 10 to 30 minutes, maybe stirring occasionally. The resulting liquid should then be strained and drunk.

Herbal remedies are now considered useful in treating central nervous system disorders, of which fibromyalgia is one. Herbal nerve tonics and stress-reducing adaptogens are particularly supportive of the nervous system.

The following two herbs are known to be useful in treating some of the symptoms of fibromyalgia.

Ginkgo biloba

Many studies have been carried out on *Ginkgo biloba,* and its effectiveness is now well documented. When used in the treatment of fibromyalgia, this herb can help maintain and support the body's circulation, particularly to the extremities (the hands and feet) and, most importantly, the brain. The advantages include better cerebral blood flow, improved tissue oxygenation, more efficient energy production and improved cognitive function in terms of concentration and short-term memory.

In a 1992 trial,[9] volunteers were given doses of 40 mg of *Ginkgo biloba* three times a day. After one month, their short-term memories had improved noticeably. In another trial,[10] 600 mg doses were given daily. The volunteers experienced even sharper reactions and better memories, without side effects, indicating improved brain functioning, all of which was judged to be due to improved circulation. *Ginkgo biloba* is, therefore, considered useful in the treatment of fibromyalgia.

St. John's wort

St. John's wort is probably the most successful natural antidepressant. Studies have shown that it works by increasing the action of the chemical serotonin (as noted earlier, people with fibromyalgia normally have low levels of available serotonin) and by inhibiting depression-promoting enzymes. Similar effects are created by the Prozac and Nardil families of orthodox antidepressants, but both have a high risk of side effects. St. John's wort, however, has the happy advantage of being virtually side-effect free. In some cases it can cause an upset stomach, but this should stop within a few days. In Germany, this herb outsells Prozac by three to one and is said to be just as effective. St. John's wort also has anti-inflammatory properties. and is believed to encourage sleep and benefit the immune system. It helps fight viral infections, too. For it to have its full effect typically takes two weeks.

Note: Because your skin may be more sensitive to the sun's rays when you are taking this herb, don't forget to use a good sunblock.

Homeopathy

The homeopathic approach to medicine is holistic—that is, the overall health of a person, their physical, emotional and psychological well being, is assessed before treatment commences. The homeopathic belief is that the whole makeup of a person determines the disorders to which they are prone, and the symptoms likely to occur. After a thorough consultation, the homeopath will offer a remedy that is compatible with the patient's symptoms as well as their temperament and characteristics. Consequently, two people with the same disorder may be offered entirely different remedies.

Homeopathic remedies are derived from plant, mineral and animal substances, which are soaked in alcohol to extract what are known as the "live" ingredients. This initial solution is then diluted many times, being vigorously shaken to add energy at each dilution. Impurities are removed and the remaining solution made up into tables, ointments, powders or suppositories. Low-dilution remedies are used for severe symptoms, while high-dilution remedies are used for milder symptoms.

Since antiquity, the homeopathic concept has been that "like cures like." The full healing abilities of this type of remedy were first recognized in the early nineteenth century when a German doctor, Samuel Hahnemann, noticed that the herbal cure for malaria—which was based on an extract of cinchona bark (quinine)—actually produced symptoms of malaria. Further tests convinced him that the production of mild symptoms caused the body to fight the disease. He went on to successfully treat malaria patients with diluted doses of cinchona bark.

Each homeopathic remedy has first been "proved" by being taken by healthy people—usually volunteer homeopaths—and the symptoms noted. The remedy is then known to be capable of curing the same symptoms in an ill person. The whole idea of "proving" and using homeopathic remedies can be difficult to understand, especially as it is exactly the opposite of how conventional medicines operate. For example, in homeopathy, a patient who has a cold with a runny nose would be treated with a remedy that would produce a runny nose in a healthy patient. Conventional medicine, on the other hand, would provide something that dries up the nose in a healthy or ill person.

Nowadays, a homeopathic remedy can be formulated to aid virtually every disorder. Although remedies are safe and non-addictive, occasionally the patient's symptoms may briefly worsen. This is known as a "healing crisis" and is usually short-lived. It is actually a good indication that the remedy is working well.

You should visit a homeopath if you have a medical problem that is not getting better or if you are constantly swapping one set of symptoms for another. It is a common misconception that you can just pop along to your local pharmacist, look up your particular complaint on the homeopathic remedy chart and begin taking the remedy. If only it were that simple. Homeopathic training takes several years, and a lot of knowledge and experience is required before practitioners can decide the correct remedies for complaints other than the very superficial. Also, as mentioned earlier, what works for one person will not always work for another, so a proper consultation is essential.

Selecting an appropriate remedy is only part of the procedure, however. The homeopath will also evaluate patient reaction to ascertain what, if any, further treatment is necessary. People who use prescribed homeopathic remedies generally notice a rapid improvement in their condition.

Hydrotherapy

I thought it appropriate here to mention a self-help therapy that can be done at home. As most of us are already aware, a long soak in a hot bath is profoundly relaxing. It also has a wonderfully calming effect on the central nervous system.

Even more soothing, surprisingly, is a long soak in a bath as close as possible to body temperature 98.6°F. For best results, the bathwater should cover your shoulders and the longer you are immersed, the better you will feel. For comfort, place a folded towel behind your head. The water should provide adequate support, though, as a body in water weighs only a quarter of its normal weight. Keep the temperature of the water as constant as possible by regularly adding hot water from the tap.

Hypnotherapy

Hypnotherapy may be described as psychotherapy using hypnosis. However, there is still no acceptable definition of the actual state of hypnosis. It is commonly described as an altered state of consciousness, lying somewhere between being awake and asleep. People under hypnosis are aware of their surroundings, yet their minds are, to a large extent, under the control of the hypnotherapist. People under hypnosis also seem to pass control of their actions, as well as a portion of their thoughts, to the hypnotherapist. You may have seen people under hypnosis on TV, acting out a role. At the time they are absorbed in what they have been "told" to do—often instigated by a specific "trigger" word—but immediately afterward they wonder what on earth they were up to. Their behavior had been dictated, to a certain degree, by the hypnotist. Hypnotherapy is about the therapist using this power for therapeutic purposes rather than entertainment.

Hypnotherapy is performed by putting the patient into a "trance." By the early nineteenth century, some physicians were using hypnotism—then called "mesmerism"—to perform pain-free operations. The majority of the medical profession were highly skeptical, believing the patients to have been either taught or paid to show no pain. Not until the last two decades did hypnotherapy become an accepted form of therapy.

Nowadays, a hypnotherapist takes a full psychological and physiological history of each patient, then slowly talks them into a trance state. The therapist can use either direct suggestion—by indicating that the patient's pain, for example, will notably lessen—or begin to explore the root cause of any tension, anxiety or depression. Of course, where fibromyalgia is concerned, physical pain is present as well as certain psychological problems. Hypnotherapy can, therefore, be very helpful.

Hypnotherapists have found that when, in chronic pain conditions, the level of tension is lowered, many of the physical symptoms are also greatly reduced. Some experts in the field believe that the main purpose of hypnotherapy is to aid relaxation, reduce tension and increase the person's confidence and ability to cope with problems.

One common fear is that the therapist may implant dangerous suggestions or extract improper personal information while the patient is in a trance. I can only say that a trance is not a wholly stable condition. Patients can come out of it at any time—particularly if they are asked to do or say anything they would not even contemplate when awake. Malpractice would only have to be detected once to ruin the therapist's entire career. Still, if you are at all worried, go to a recommended hypnotherapist.

Massage

Massage therapy was one of the earliest treatments used by humankind. It enjoyed only average popularity, however, until the nineteenth century, when a Swedish athlete found that a combination of massage and exercise greatly relaxed muscles and joints. This therapy became far more popular when, in 1970, George Dowling's *The Massage Book* (Penguin) was published. It introduced the concept of a holistic approach to the whole technique of massage. Nowadays, the emotional and psychological state, as well as the physical state, are assessed at the initial consultation.

A good massage helps a person feel relaxed, both physically and mentally. It is useful in treating depression and anxiety as well as headaches, stiffness, muscle pain and circulatory disorders. It is not, however, appropriate for people suffering inflammation of the veins (phlebitis), varicose veins or thrombosis. Your GP will tell you whether or not you are a suitable candidate and may even supply details of a qualified therapist.

The massage itself consists of the actions of stroking, drumming, kneading and/or friction (sometimes called "pressure"). These methods may be used separately or in combination, depending on the patient's symptoms. For fibromyalgics, it is advisable, first of all, to inquire whether or not the practitioner is familiar with the condition. Stroking and gentle kneading techniques may be acceptable, but drumming and friction massage might aggravate your symptoms. For some sufferers, even a light pressure massage can be sufficient to induce severe pain. It is important, therefore, that you speak up if the therapist begins to hurt you.

After a request by the Fibromyalgia Network USA for feedback on the subject of massage therapy, 300 letters were received. An overwhelming majority praised the treatment, many saying that if their budgets allowed, they would have weekly therapy. Because deep massage techniques were often too painful to tolerate, however, most respondents began with some form of "light touch" therapy. People with severe symptoms started out with a partial body massage (neck, shoulders and back), many leading up to a full-body massage as their toleration increased.

Most times, if you want a massage you have to travel to a massage clinic, but some practitioners make home visits. You will be asked to undress, leaving on only your panties or briefs. If this makes you feel uneasy, you should insist that another person be present. Nowadays, practitioners often combine treatment with aromatherapy, acupuncture or reflexology.

After therapy, many people report an increase in function and a reduction of fatigue. Fibromyalgics should rest afterward to make sure that loosened muscles do not immediately re-knot. It is unwise to carry a heavy load of shopping home just because you feel better, for example. Where muscles have successfully been released, you may have soreness for up to two days afterward. Rest will help ensure that a delayed pain response is minimized.

For sore post-massage muscles, place an ice pack (gel packs that can be both frozen and heated can be purchased at most drug stores) on the affected areas. Alternating between cold and heat can be even more beneficial. Taking a warm bath later that evening, maybe with a teaspoonful of Epsom salts, can also help reduce any post-massage soreness.

For those who feel competent and wish to massage someone at home, ensure that the room is warm and peaceful and lay the recipient on a comfortable but firm surface. A pillow placed beneath the upper torso may help to relax the upper back. Massage oil (aromatherapy oils are good) makes the act of massage easier, and hand movements should be smooth, gentle and continuous. Continue the therapy for two or three minutes only, to ensure there are no unwelcome after effects. If all is well, gradually increase the length of the sessions.

Your local library should carry several books on the subject of massage techniques, many of them including advice on self-massage. Or you could purchase an electric massager, which you may be able to use yourself. To ease discomfort in more inaccessible areas, ask a friend or partner to help out.

Reflexology

Reflexology, an ancient oriental therapy, has only relatively recently been adopted in the Western world. It works on the principle that the body is divided into different energy zones, represented in different parts of the feet, all of which can be exploited in the prevention and treatment of any disorder.

Reflexologists have identified 10 energy channels, which run from the toes and extend to the fingers and the top of the head. Each channel relates to a particular body zone, and to the organs in that zone. For example, the big toe relates to the head—the brain, sinus area, neck, pituitary glands, eyes and ears. By applying pressure to the appropriate terminal in the form of a specialized massage, a practitioner can determine which energy pathways are blocked. Minute lumps—like crystalline deposits—detected beneath the skin are then broken down by steady pressure. The theory is that the deposits are absorbed into the body's waste disposal system and eliminated in sweat or urine, hence restoring the correct energy flow.

Experts in this type of manipulative therapy claim that reflexology aids the removal of waste products and blockages within the energy channels, improving circulation and the functioning of the glands. Reflexology is certainly relaxing—indeed, many patients fall asleep during therapy. Because my own feet are so ticklish, I felt I had cause to worry before my first reflexology session—I could imagine myself involuntarily kicking the therapist in the teeth! Fortunately, I quickly found that the sensations were pleasurable and I was able to relax. I must say, I was surprised to note how accurate the therapist was in detecting my own "indispositions."

Many therapists prefer to take down a full case history before commencing treatment. Each session takes up to 45 minutes (the preliminary session will take longer) and you will be treated either sitting in a chair or lying down, depending on both therapist and patient.

6

Pain and Stress Management

*I'd love to be able to pour out my heart when someone asks how
I am! I'd love to be able to say how scared and useless I feel!
But I don't dare. I'd be thought a self-pitying wimp! . . . Oh, if only
I could find some way of managing all the emotions whirling
around in my head, of getting people to believe in me!*

Fibromyalgia can affect every area of our lives. In the early stages of the
illness, we are often beset by fears for the future, anxieties about our
effectiveness as "functioning" human beings and even doubts about
our sanity. Negative feedback from others is also a major source of
upset. However, given time, education and self-awareness training, we
can gradually adapt to the illness, finding ways to effectively cope with
the pain, stress and reactions of others. Just as importantly, we can learn
to focus on the present, recapturing feelings of achievement by acquir-
ing new interests and maybe even a new, more fulfilling career. All
these things go a long way toward enhancing the quality of life.

A Chronic Illness

Many people fail to appreciate that any chronic illness—fibromyalgia
included—creates problems within the mind as well as the body.
Feelings of unreality, vulnerability, guilt, uselessness, fear and being out
of control taint our dealings with others and can be incredibly difficult
to shake off.

"I feel so unsure of myself"

The complexity of fibromyalgia can give rise to much self-doubt, particularly in the early months/years of the illness. When we have pain that, like a ghost, mysteriously transfers from one area to another, when diagnostic tests indicate that everything is fine and when doctors as well as those closest to us stare suspiciously as we describe our unusual symptoms, we may start to wonder if our problems really are of the mind rather than the body!

The fear of mental illness is very real in us all, but to believe it to be a possibility is terrifying. Losing control of our minds means losing connection with ourselves and the world we live in. Ironically, threats to our rationality can cause emotional problems—stress, anxiety and depression—all of which are far from helpful to our overall state of mind!

Doctors who fail to understand the effects of chronic illness on the individual—especially where there is no validating diagnosis—invariably amplify these problems. Even after the diagnosis, they can compound the situation by failing to provide information about the disease, neglecting to offer guidance on self-help coping techniques and omitting to outline different treatment options. Unable to cope with the patient's ensuing despair, the doctor is then likely to refer the patient to a psychologist. Sadly, this only serves to endorse the patient's suspicions that they have mental problems.

It is a fact that where long-term illness defeats diagnosis, doctors often suspect the problem to be psychological in origin. Consequently, even though a correct diagnosis may eventually be given, one of stress, anxiety, depression or even a type of neurosis will remain in the patient's medical records, coloring prospective treatment choices and maybe swaying opinion in a future diagnosis.

"I feel so vulnerable"

Vulnerability is a natural human condition. We all need people to love us; we all crave the affirmation of others. To a large extent, we are all dependent on others, measuring their responses in order to reassure ourselves that we are worthwhile human beings, that we are indeed loveable. When we are chronically ill, as well as feeling unattractive, we believe we have little to offer the people around us and so fear we are no longer loveable.

Feelings of vulnerability will always be present in chronic illness, but we can defeat the worst of them by looking less to outsiders for affirmation. We all have inner strengths and particular talents, many of which we may not realize. Yet, if we waited for others to point them out we would likely be waiting forever!

Your particular forte may be in planning and organizing or problem-solving or handling finances—not necessarily out of the family setting. You may be an authority on steam engines, an inspired cook, a good listener, a talented artist, an excellent singer, a diligent student, a competent driver . . . so do not underestimate yourself!

"I feel so guilty"

Feelings of guilt are common in chronic illness. It is natural to want to lay the blame for falling ill at someone's door, and many of us imagine we ourselves must have done something very wrong to deserve such retribution. Blaming either ourselves or others, though, is pointless. Life is a lottery. Some people are rich, some poor; some clever, some not so clever; some fall ill, some remain healthy. That's just the way it is.

After learning that improvement lies mainly in your hands, you may feel guilty if you are making no real progress. However, assuming you have tried to help yourself, there is probably a sound reason for your failure. For example, you may have been unable to find information about exactly how to help yourself, be held back by additional health problems or not have allowed sufficient time for any improvements to show.

Pain flare-ups are a perpetual threat in fibromyalgia. Although they can result from "outside" influences—the weather, a fall, a family crisis—it is likely that a chosen activity caused the exacerbation of pain. So you feel guilty. Viewing a flare-up as a "painful" learning experience may be some consolation. You attempted to clean the oven, but afterwards you were rigid with pain. It was a hard lesson but you learned that cleaning the cooker is bad for you!

Guilt also arises when we feel we are a burden on our families. We feel bad about their extra workload and because their free time is now so limited. When fibromyalgics need "full-time" caregivers, it is important that the carers have time to themselves, that they retain certain interests and have occasional time off. The knowledge that they are enjoying their lives regardless of your ill health and limitations—which, of course, they have a perfect right to do—should help you feel far less guilty.

"I feel so afraid"

Of course we are afraid when we have an illness for which there is, as yet, no absolute cure. Our fears tend to center on the future and what will become of us. We are afraid of being in constant pain, of deteriorating further, of becoming entirely dependent on others, of the long-term effects of medication, of losing all our friends . . . the list is endless.

Chronic illness exerts profound effects on the individual. It is not always easy to be cheerful and bright when you have a cold, never mind a painful, energy-sapping illness you can see no end to. At least you know that the cold will soon pass, at least you can tell yourself that your spirits will then be restored. As a fibromyalgic, you cannot comfort yourself in this way.

However, in most cases of fibromyalgia, the fear of the unknown abates with time. We learn we can take pleasure from family life, enjoy social occasions, take up interests and hobbies and be of use to others. Most importantly, we learn that our condition really can improve—there is no evidence to suggest that fibromyalgia is a degenerative disease. In realizing that the majority of our fears are unfounded, we can get on with our lives more cheerfully.

"I feel so useless"

Fibromyalgia is, without doubt, a limiting condition. After the onset of the illness, tasks that were once accomplished with ease either have to be performed with caution or dropped altogether. More often than not, many tasks around the house have to be allocated to other family members or to a paid cleaner. Onlookers may quip, "Lucky you—having someone else do all the hard work!" They don't realize you would give anything to be able to clean the house thoroughly each and every day.

It is the same with many of the activities you previously enjoyed—and not necessarily ones requiring much effort. Many sufferers are unable to tilt their heads to read or write (myself included, although I am now able to type for an hour and a half a day). Knitting, sewing, sketching, even such trivial tasks as filling tea kettle, can cause similar problems and may have to be set aside for the present.

Don't give up hope of ever again being able to do the things you enjoyed, though. The heaviest and most "stretching" of tasks may be permanently out of your scope, but other pleasures (and tasks) can be achieved given time, patience and by the employment of pain and stress management strategies. The early months/years of illness are by far the most forbidding, but later you may find you are able to do many of the things you thought you had to set aside forever.

"I feel so out of control"

Having little control over your fibromyalgia is frightening, but as with many other problems, this feeling is exaggerated during the early months/years. Attempts at regaining a sense of control by, for example, dishing out orders from your sick bed or interfering in other people's lives are not a good idea, however!

In time, we generally evolve our own coping strategies—many we may not even be aware of—and learn how to master certain problem situations. We may even end up having more control over our lives than beforehand! For example, we can learn to control the way we talk to and respond to others, train our minds to focus on the present instead of the future, discipline ourselves to take disappointments in our stride and control our viewpoints, developing a more positive, realistic approach to life.

An Invisible Illness

The thoughtlessness and distrust of others creates difficulties for all sufferers of invisible illness. Even our nearest and dearest can say something hurtful during a careless moment. The reason? Simply because they cannot measure our pain, fatigue, anxiety and, for a moment, have failed to bring to mind all we have told them.

When the greater part of their behavior indicates their concern, however, we can forgive that momentary lapse. We get upset, though, when others fail to make the same effort, when they show no interest in how we feel or when they interpret our "behavior" as weakness. Getting upset serves no useful purpose, however. It only increases the tension in our already painful muscles; it only amplifies stress.

Most people are spurred into activity at the sight of, say, a traffic accident. Instinctively forming a team, "onlookers" each play a part in trying to help the injured, making them as comfortable as possible, warning and diverting approaching traffic and alerting the emergency services. Urgency and compassion galvanize them into action. In some instances, onlookers go so far as to put their own lives at risk in their determination to help a person—or even an animal—in trouble. However, those same people are rarely galvanized into action when the crisis is not manifest, when someone suffering from an invisible illness complains of pain or exhaustion.

"Why do people distrust what I say?"

Suspicion arises when, as in fibromyalgia, pain cannot be quantified. Onlookers are unable to see the pain, nor can they see any of the hodge-podge of symptoms from which the sufferer is complaining. In fact, they have never heard of fibromyalgia, so how can it be that bad? Pain that mysteriously travels from one area to another—stomach problems and itching one day, exhaustion and migraine the next—what kind of an illness is that? You have to admit, fibromyalgia is not the easiest of conditions for others to accept.

The people who are trusting and compassionate by nature are usually the first to accept invisible illness in others; they are often the first to offer a friendly ear as well as practical help and advice. Those who spend time with fibromyalgics gradually see for themselves how limited their lives have become, how they have ceased activities they formerly enjoyed. That is down to what is visible.

It is human nature to be suspicious and, sadly, some onlookers are quick to tag fibromyalgics as soft, inadequate and attention-seekers. Being judged in this way is upsetting, especially when in most instances the reverse is actually true. Experts now believe that the majority of people with fibromyalgia play down their symptoms. Among the myriad reasons for this, past unfortunate experiences with others leads the field.

Few of you will not have endured boredom, embarrassment or disbelief as you attempted to explain your symptoms to someone asking about your health. As a result, you may have got into the habit of muttering, "I'm not too bad, thanks" or "A bit better today . . ." but, unfortunately, playing down a little-known condition such as fibromyalgia can actually come across as indecision about whether or not you are feeling ill at all! Furthermore, being uncertain of your limitations and giving vague, half-hearted responses only serve to moisten any seeds of doubt already planted in the other person's mind.

It sounds like you can't win, doesn't it? Conveying the nature, severity and complexity of fibromyalgia is, without doubt, incredibly hard work. However, if you are not straightforward, open and brief— listeners get bored when people harp on about their illness—certain people around you may never understand.

"How can I make people understand?"

Sarcastic and derisive remarks from others can chip away at your confidence. Therefore, they should not pass unchallenged. Standing up for yourself is not easy, but doing so can have a releasing effect—the opposite of how you feel when you fake indifference or clam up and walk away. In such instances, you may end up feeling hurt, offended, and very resentful. Your most intense feeling, however, is likely to be that of anger— toward the other person and yourself, for allowing yourself to be hurt.

For example, if your partner were to complain "I do all the housework while you do nothing," I suggest you respond "I'm trying as hard as I can, but when I have a flare-up, everything I do makes me worse. I know it seems unfair when you're stuck with all the housework. . . . Maybe it will help you to know that seeing you so busy upsets me, too. I really do appreciate your efforts, though. Perhaps we should learn to put up with a bit of dust and clutter." If the initial comment was made during a heated exchange, you could answer, "That's a hurtful thing to say. I may be doing very little, but it's not my fault. I'd like to talk this through when we're calmer."

When family members are consistently skeptical of your condition—no matter what words or manner you employ—you may be so hurt you consider cutting yourself off from them completely. If their condemnations of you border on the fanatical, then this is perhaps your only choice. Otherwise, you would be best advised to keep steadily hammering away at your case, remembering to bring all unfair comments to their attention.

It may help you to know that when someone close remains deaf to your assertions of ill health, it is often because they can't face the fact that their child/partner/parent/sibling/best friend is very ill. The only way they can deal with your illness is to refuse to believe in it. In effect, they cope by not coping. However, that is their problem, not yours. Don't ever give up on them, for almost everything changes with time.

Sadly, people outside your immediate circle of friends/relatives are often capable of being as cutting as the people close to you. Again, they have no right to hurt you, and should not get away with it. Your best weapons here are words that make them think. For example, a person who asks mockingly, "Are we any better today?" could be answered with, "Is there something on your mind? If so, just say it. . . . If you really are concerned about my health, thank you. The truth is my back is hurting terribly and I don't know how I'll manage to get home."

Fibromyalgics frequently face remarks such as, "I noticed you went shopping last Saturday. I thought you weren't able to walk far!" or "I saw you at the club on Sunday. You must be feeling better!" In such situations, replies could be along the lines of "Yes, I did manage to get out last weekend. I have good days and bad. Even though I was feeling better, I still had to spend two days in bed afterward."

"Why have I lost so many friends?"

As you may already have discovered, having fibromyalgia leaves you in little doubt as to who your real friends are. The "friends" who are offended when you break an appointment, the "friends" who are unconvinced when you explain that, yes, you were able to have a night out with them last week, but you feel too ill to go out tonight and worse still the "friends" who complain that you have let them down again are really not worth your precious energies. Their negative input into your life is detrimental to your confidence as well as to your health.

Guilt is a natural consequence of letting people down. The feeling is amplified when you regularly renege on pre-arranged activities. The ill feeling you know it engenders in others may spur you into attempting activities you know will make you suffer. You may turn up at the next social event despite feeling particularly "delicate," despite knowing that doing so may provoke a flare-up. Placing yourself at risk in this way is really not worth the fact that you have temporarily assuaged your guilt.

What about the "friends" who, after you have been unable to socialize as before, have gradually dropped out of your life? Can you honestly say they were true friends? Wouldn't a true friend make allowances for your illness? Wouldn't a true friend try to understand what you are going through?

"Why do people make me feel so upset?"

Even if everyone were charming and accepting around us, fibromyalgia would be a frustrating, upsetting, anger-making business. The reactions of some of the people in our lives only serve to intensify these feelings. We know the condemnation someone who is frequently off sick from work receives. We may even have previously thought badly of someone who regularly complained of ill health. We know that society in general is contemptuous of both mental and physical weakness. When we become ill, all this knowledge seems to form a tight ball in our heads. It only takes one careless comment and we either explode in rage or feel so upset and despairing we want to hide ourselves away.

Without doubt, some people are incredibly insensitive. We may feel we are always on our guard, dreading the remark that will send us into a whirl of anger or spiralling to the depths of despair. Sadly, chronic invisible illness lays us wide open to the misunderstandings of others. As I said earlier, hurtful comments should always be pointed out. If the perpetrator appears contrite, go on to briefly explain just how the illness affects you.

Dealing with Negative Thinking

Much negative thinking arises from early conditioning. For example, the children of parents who consistently make the same type of comment often grow up with similar basic attitudes. If a woman regularly scoffs at weakness or if her husband or partner repeatedly declares that incompetence is unforgivable, their children have a fair chance of growing up believing this way of thinking is valid and proper.

When people frequently voice negative thoughts, it usually means they are afraid of the very thing about which they are being negative. The mother who decries weakness does it because she secretly fears she is weak. It is the same with the father who denounces incompetence. His attitude stems from deep-seated doubts about his own competence. When their offspring copy these attitudes in adulthood, condemning weakness and incompetence as well as displaying other negative viewpoints, this, too, stems from inherent beliefs that they are lacking in many ways.

Our mindsets—that is, approaching life with an attitude of either trust or distrust, enthusiasm or depression, self-assurance or timidity, anxiety or serenity and so on—usually arise from childhood conditioning. Our automatic thoughts are, therefore, determined by whatever mindsets are built into our character, controlling our behavior in any given situation. For example, when planning a birthday party, a person with a depressive mindset would dread the "big day," worrying that few guests would even turn up. A person with an enthusiastic mindset, on the other hand, would eagerly await the party, sure of its success. A person with a trustful mindset would take "That sweater's a bit small for you" as a caring remark and happily change into something that fitted better. A person with a distrustful mindset, on the other hand, would take it as a criticism of their weight, the sweater, their choice of clothes or all these put together!

Irrational feelings

Negative mindsets invariably produce irrational feelings about ourselves and these feelings often become self-fulfilling prophesies. For example, thinking "I will never be any good with money" stops us trying to be good with money. "I will never make anyone happy" stops us trying to make anyone happy and, concerning our ill health, "I am no fun to have around any more" makes us stop trying to be good-humored about the situation. These irrational feelings determine our behavior. Unfortunately, chronic illness is often the spark that sets irrational feelings blazing out of control.

However, these feelings can be turned around. We can learn a new, more positive approach to life. First, however, we need to acknowledge our irrational thoughts and feelings for what they are, and for the behavior they induce. Family celebrations commonly provoke feelings of anxiety in people with fibromyalgia. Actually writing down our negative thoughts and feelings, and really analyzing them, can make the fact they are irrational crystal clear, it makes us more aware.

Here is an example of possible irrational thoughts and feelings prior to a family party.

Situation: Family party

Irrational thoughts: "I will be a real wet blanket. No one will want to talk to me. I will put a dampener on the whole event."

Irrational feelings: "I will be a real wet blanket. No one will want to talk to me. I will put a dampener on the whole event. I will then feel sad, hurt and alienated. I will hate myself for being such a misery."

This example illustrates just how irrational chronic illness can make us at times. Yet, if we do not analyze them, the potential repercussions can be staggering. In the example above, you may end up talking yourself into staying at home, experiencing a mixture of self-pity, guilt and even self-loathing. Your decision could even cause an argument with your partner . . . .

The example also reveals a common tendency for people to worry about something that may never happen. If it is Wednesday and you are in the middle of a flare-up, don't fret about a party scheduled for the weekend! You are hardly likely to be well enough to attend and your family should be made aware of that fact. However, if you are no worse than usual, then, realistically, staying at home is hardly the answer. No matter how dire your "normal" condition for the sake of sanity, you need to have a life; you need to be with others occasionally, so you need to make an extra effort every now and again. Given sufficient advance planning, certain events really can be managed effectively. Whether your symptoms are severe or not, backing out of events or activities you may have enjoyed can leave you feeling angry with yourself, furious with your illness and resentful that everyone else is in good health!

I was taught to record my thoughts and feelings before a troublesome event, and doing so always helps me. Try it and see if it helps you, too. Assuming, then, that you are no worse than usual, try to write down your assumptions about your presence at the party. Now look objectively at what you have written. Are your thoughts and feelings reasonable? No doubt you would feel like a wet blanket if you sat with a face as long as a fiddle and made no effort to talk to anyone! Could you really be so rude that you would avoid talking with people? Are your relatives really so antisocial that they would disregard you?

When we challenge negative feelings in such a way, the reality of the situation soon becomes apparent. People make an effort to be friendly at family gatherings. Your fellow guests are people you know well. Common ground can always be found, should you wish to look for it.

So, you have re-evaluated and subsequently banished one set of negative thoughts, only to find it is swiftly replaced by another. You have decided to attend the party, but now you are worrying about coping with pain in company. Will the pain totally consume you? Will you burst into tears? Will everyone think you pathetic?

Although it is normal to worry about coping with pain when you are out of your usual environment, your worries may be somewhat distorted due to your fears. Writing them down helps you see them in a more detached light. Below, I have expanded on the example above by incorporating a column listing possible solutions.

Situation: "I will be in a lot of pain at the party."

Irrational thoughts: "I will be unable to cope with the pain. I will feel as if I could cry. I will get angry and accuse everyone of not caring."

Irrational feelings: "People will think me weak and stupid. They will hate me for spoiling the occasion. I will then feel angry with myself."

Solution: "I will take painkillers before leaving and take more with me for later. I'll ask to lie down if I start to feel bad."

Here, irrational feelings are seen for what they are and possible solutions are considered. Other solutions may include choosing the most supportive chair there, asking for a hot water bottle for your back or explaining in advance that you may have to leave early. After all, looking for realistic ways in which to ease a difficult situation is far more helpful than immersing yourself in worries that get you nowhere. More importantly, it can help you cope with some degree of pain.

You may then find yourself assailed by further worries. You have planned to ask if you may lie down, but, when the time comes, you feel anxious about actually doing so. Surely your hosts will think you feeble and demanding. Surely everyone will stare and whisper behind your back. This again is irrational thinking, and as you obviously won't always be able to write your feelings down, you should mentally consider what you need to do. In this instance, all you can do—unless you want to risk incurring the usual thoughts of self-loathing and self-pity, on top of a certain increase in pain—is ask.

From personal experience, I can honestly say that people are only too willing to assist when asked directly. Often they haven't been sure what to say, but when you ask for help, it takes the pressure off them. They will likely then want to know whether the bedroom is warm enough, the bed firm enough, the pillows soft enough. . . . If they do scowl and make a comment to the effect that you are making a fuss—and in all my years of asking others for help regarding my fibromyalgia, I have never come across anyone who has—it says a lot more about their nature than yours!

Helping Others to Understand

In attempting to help the people you care about understand your fibromyalgia, you should try to speak clearly and openly. Brevity also has a positive impact, as has being honest about how you feel.

Speaking openly

Before endeavoring to describe your feelings, you first need to focus on how you actually do feel. It may be difficult to admit you feel guilty, frustrated, angry, useless, vulnerable . . . even to yourself. Sharing your feelings with others is even more difficult, yet it is an important step toward halting the problems those feelings can cause. In your need to be understood by others, however, you should be wary of making assumptions about how they feel about you.

Speaking to others in the following way is sure to cause offense: "I get so upset when you think I'm exaggerating" or "I don't believe you really care about me, and that makes me feel so hopeless" or "I'm losing confidence because you treat me as if I'm not trying to help myself." Such comments will likely be seen as accusations; they may even provoke a quarrel. Speaking directly of your "emotional problems"—without implying that the other person is contributing to those problems—will incline them to take your comments more seriously. It should also encourage them to be more thoughtful in future. Before undertaking to speak openly of your feelings, however, the following list of considerations should be taken into account.

- *Be sure you have interpreted the other person's behavior correctly.* For example, you may view your mother bringing you a basket of fruit and vegetables as a criticism of your diet when, in truth, it is a goodwill gesture, just to show she cares! You have a perfect right to interpret the words or actions of others in whatever way you wish, but that interpretation is not necessarily reality. In fact, it is amazing how wrong we often are in our perceptions of what others think and feel.

- *Be sure you are specific in recalling another person's behavior.* For example, "You never understand how exhausted I get," is far more inflammatory than "You didn't seem to understand yesterday, when I told you how exhausted I felt."

- *Be sure that what you are about to say is what you really mean.* For example, statements such as, "Everyone thinks you're insensitive," or "We all think you've got an attitude problem," besides being inflammatory, are very unfair. We have no way of knowing that "everyone" is of the same opinion. The use of the depersonalized "everyone," "we" or "us"—often said in the hope of deflecting the listener's anger—can cause more hurt and anger than if the criticism was direct and personal.

It's easy to see how others can misunderstand or take offense when we fail to communicate effectively. However, changing the habits of a lifetime is difficult. It means analyzing our thoughts before rearranging them into speech. We are rewarded for our efforts, however, when people start to listen, when they cease to be annoyed as we carefully explain an area they don't fully understand. Once we have stopped trying to improve others, we can begin to focus on improving ourselves and our own situations.

Dealing with your co-workers

If you are managing to work and cope with fibromyalgia at the same time, well done! Exceptions for chronic ill health in the workplace generally have to be fought for. Even when your boss is tolerant, your co-workers often are not.

If your fibromyalgia is not yet acknowledged at work, be prepared for a struggle, but never be tempted to cover up your health-related shortcomings. Those who do so are rarely shown leniency. In fact, unless you are able to communicate the nature of your illness and how it affects your performance, you are liable to be condemned as slow and inefficient—especially by co-workers who are convinced you are not pulling your weight.

Strangely enough, given sufficient information about the illness, employers can be more sympathetic than some fellow employees. Your exclusion from certain duties can prompt certain co-workers to make snide remarks. Whether these remarks are related to jealousy, resentment or distrust or are simply made because you are an easy target when they are having a bad day, they are cruel and unjust, so should not be tolerated!

The thought of objecting to an unfair accusation, particularly when you are at a low ebb, may seem daunting. However, besides being the only means of getting through to some people, it also helps you maintain your self-esteem. For example, a co-worker may remark, "You look fine. I'm sure you're using your illness to get out of doing the filing!" Whether the tone is lighthearted or not, the content is hostile and undeserved. Failing to respond—maybe because you are too angry, too hurt, or simply too tired—only serves to confirm their opinion. Your answer should be a firm, "I resent that. I'm glad you think I look okay, but I don't use my illness as an excuse, and I don't have to prove myself to you." The co-worker will usually apologize at this point and may even confess, "I suppose I just don't understand your illness." Here is your chance to explain more about fibromyalgia.

Whenever others appear to be in a receptive frame of mind, try to grasp the opportunity to explain your condition. Your symptoms may best be understood when you equate them to something within the listener's experience. For instance, "The fatigue can feel like the flu" or, to someone who has suffered sports injuries, "The pain in my shoulder is like that of a torn ligament," helps them see exactly how it is for you. Descriptive analogies can be effective, too (so long as you don't go over the top)—for example, "The pain is like needles piercing the base of my neck," "It feels like my back's been pummelled by a boxer," make the listener really think. Explain, too, the most troublesome of the additional symptoms from which you suffer, making sure to emphasize that they are all elements of your fibromyalgia. The more information you can feed to the people around you, the more likely they are to digest it.

Remember, too, that we should not expect everyone we encounter to be openly friendly, just as we may not be openly friendly toward everyone we meet. Some personalities just don't mix. Only in accepting this fact can you help yourself disregard those who refuse to listen.

Getting the best from your doctor

You may have suffered alarming symptoms for several months, expecting them to subside any day, but, instead, the mysteriously shifting pain persists, the headaches and fatigue have worsened and you have become sensitive to certain foods, certain chemicals, cold, damp and light. Feeling let down and confused when sympathetic ears become difficult to find, you turn to your doctor. You crave answers, but you worry that the doctor, like your family and friends, will think you are imagining it all. It is upsetting when people close to you are distrustful, but professional distrust is devastating.

Doctors are frequently baffled by the unusual symptoms of fibromyalgia and misdiagnosis—maybe one of anxiety, stress, depression, hysteria or some kind of neurosis—is not unusual. The misdiagnosis may be confirmed in your doctor's mind when you reply to the questions "Would you say you're a worrier?" "How are you and your partner getting on?" "Are you happy at work?" with a "Since the illness took hold, I have been eaten up with worry, suffered relationship problems and had difficulties performing at work and getting along with co-workers." The outcome may be a course of antidepressants, plus advice to the effect that you need a break from routine.

Few fibromyalgics have not had difficult dealings with doctors somewhere along the line. Yet, if your relationship with your doctor is not good, your health can suffer unnecessarily.

Poor communication on the part of the patient may, in the first place, lead to misdiagnosis. The following are examples of what can go wrong.

- For fear of being prejudged, patients tend to censor their descriptions of certain symptoms, such as anxiety, depression and so on.
- In their desperation to secure a diagnosis, patients may bombard—and therefore confuse—the doctor with a multitude of outwardly unrelated symptoms.
- In deference to the doctor's lack of time, patients may describe only their main symptom(s), omitting those that may otherwise help the doctor to arrive at an accurate conclusion.
- Eager to emphasize that they are neither lazy nor malingering, patients may incorrectly interpret the doctor's questions. For example, if the question "How are your stamina levels?" comes up, the patient may declare, "I've never been one for sitting around. I've always had an active life." The patient thereby frustrates the doctor's attempts to draw a clearer picture.

In order to secure a prompt and accurate diagnosis, you must:
- give your doctor a full and precise description of your symptoms;
- be sure you have understood the questions before replying;
- take care to speak clearly.

Moreover, try not to forget that doctors can only work within the confines of what they have been taught—evaluating symptoms in a scientific manner and looking to specific disorders as a result of your answers to the questions. Finally, I know it's difficult, but try not to expect immediate answers.

Remember, too, that your doctor is only human. Your attitude may sway the conclusion arrived at. For example, if you are apologetic, in response the doctor may think you are imagining some of your symptoms. If you are angry with the doctor, the doctor may feel hurt and/or irritated.

As there is always a risk of a personality clash between a doctor and you, seek a doctor with whom you feel comfortable. Doctors have to maintain professional distance, but when you find one who is open-minded and understanding, hang on to him or her.

Adjusting Your Expectations

Thinking about the future is a natural human characteristic. We enjoy looking forward to vacations, holidays and other forthcoming events; we need to look ahead and project possible outcomes before we can make any kind of decision. However, when that future is clouded by the pain and fear that comes with chronic illness, we are plagued by compelling "What if . . ." questions. The bleak and hopeless years we visualize as our future appear beyond our control, yet they can haunt our waking hours as well as our dreams.

Pain will always induce anxiety, as it is hard not to fear a pain-filled future. However, looking ahead in fear is counterproductive. The first step toward conquering the inclination to worry about what may or may not happen is to tell yourself that it does no good. Controlling your thinking is far from easy, but it can be achieved. When the bleak visions loom, try to distract yourself either by turning your mind to something pleasant or, fibromyalgia withstanding, doing something requiring concentration. After such "visions" have been staved off on a regular basis, the propensity toward that type of thinking will gradually decrease.

Living in the present

People with fibromyalgia need all their resources to handle the present. A calm and contented now is more emotionally nourishing than a mind reeling with the upsets the future may or may not hold. In the same way, cherishing the moment is preferable to letting it slip by unappreciated because we are too busy thinking ahead. How many of us look forward to seeing a film, band, recital or play, but don't think to enjoy the journey there? How many of us look forward to summer, forgetting to appreciate spring? It is the same with numerous things in our lives.

"However," you may ask, "is it possible for chronic pain sufferers to master the art of living in the present?" As people with fibromyalgia, of necessity, have to always remember to pace themselves, finding enjoyable yet untaxing leisure interests is essential. After all, why sit brooding when you could be reading a gripping book, penning a poem, surfing the Internet, taking a walk or sharing views with someone close? This is the time to consider doing things you never had time for before. If, for example, assembling a model railway was a childhood dream you never managed to fulfill or if you always toyed with the idea of learning to play the piano, but never quite got around to it, this is your opportunity—fibromyalgia permitting.

Making the most of now

When you need to rest all day in anticipation of an evening out, it is important that you enjoy the day as well. Okay, so you dare not risk tackling housework, or going into town, but there is sure to be something agreeable with which you can occupy yourself in the meantime. This is your chance to select that new jacket from your catalog, update your stamp collection, muse over last year's holiday photos or simply watch that new comedy video.

Those of you who dare not risk even sitting during the intervening hours may find lying on the sofa to read, watch TV or listen to music an acceptable alternative. At times, I need to spend several hours a day lying on my back in bed, which means that until my husband and I can afford to reinforce the bedroom ceiling, I am unable to even watch TV. Believe me, having little to do but listen to music for hours made me feel very sorry for myself—that is until I discovered books on tape. Most libraries stock a varied selection, mostly bestsellers. Give them a try. They may broaden your life, as they have mine!

Looking on the bright side

Developing a positive outlook is invaluable in fibromyalgia. It stops us dwelling on the past, helps us enjoy the present and bestows hope and conviction. When we look for something pleasing in the things we do— even chores—we can significantly lighten our load.

You may be wondering, "What could possibly be pleasing about washing dishes or peeling potatoes?" Since most of us perform these tasks by the kitchen window, they have that in their favor. While you scour the pans or wash or peel the spuds, do you consciously appreciate the world outside or are you inclined to gaze blindly out, fretting about this and that? If the latter is usually the case, try to concentrate instead on really looking at, and appreciating, your outdoor environment. Admire the manifold creations of nature, observe the inventiveness in all that is manmade; notice how people behave as they go about their daily business.

As the seasons pass, consciously appreciate the effects different weather conditions have on your environment. Even the busiest and most depressing of streets can be enhanced by bright sunshine sparkling on wet rooftops, mist gliding in graceful ribbons through the air, glassy icicles hanging from windowledges, a covering of fresh snow. Enhanced? When it's so foggy you need a searchlight to find the front gate? When it's so slippery you need spikes on your shoes?

All right, so inclement weather can create numerous problems, but why think of those problems when you're snug and warm indoors? Keep your mind on the present. Let gazing at the weather—the rain, the frost, the snow—stir your senses. Children like to stretch out a hand to feel the rain, they are awed by the sight of icicles and they are so excited by snow. Often we lose that childish appreciation when we reach adulthood, but it's never too late to recapture it! The time to worry about harsh weather conditions is only shortly before you step outside!

Accepting what you can't change

Including the weather, there are many things in life we cannot change. We can do nothing about the fact that we are either creative or practical, black or white, tall or short (or anything in between). Neither can we change the fact that we have fibromyalgia, although we can certainly improve the situation. However, acknowledging what we can't change and trying to live with it is fundamental to stress management. In accepting things as they stand, we say goodbye to a great deal of frustration.

Continuing the weather analogy, it has to be said that some of us have little choice, after assessing the situation rationally, but to virtually hibernate during a prolonged cold spell. Sadly, despite the fact that feeling distanced from the rest of the world is profoundly disheartening, you can do nothing about harsh weather.

In fine weather, and barring flare-ups, you may find it easier to get out and about. You may need help with the shopping, someone with you when you visit the museum, library, hairdresser, yard sale, but you should make the most of being able to do these things. Winter, in particular, is the time to consider taking up new interests, to think about doing things you never got around to before.

Besides offering a distraction, involving yourself in a new challenge can be infinitely rewarding. Consider playing computer games, talking to other fibromyalgia sufferers via the Internet, taking up model making, woodwork, metal work, oil painting, stencilling, photography, playing the keyboard, tapestry work, glass and china painting, picture framing, jewelry making . . . the list is endless. The selection of "things to do" in a craft shop alone is quite dazzling!

Of course, not everyone with fibromyalgia is physically able to do these things. They are merely suggestions. People who have difficulty leaning forward may be unable to sketch, paint, sew or make models; people who are unable to tilt their heads are similarly limited, as are those who are physically incapable of holding out an arm for a period of time. The challenge is to find interests to suit your capabilities, as well as ones that stimulate your imagination.

Learning to let go

When fibromyalgia takes hold, many of us have no alternative but to relinquish a lifetime's ambitions. We give up our careers, as a consequence, feel we have lost much of what gave us a sense of worth and identity. However, learning to let go of what we can no longer do—possibly looking to a new, less ambitious but equally fulfilling career and searching out new interests to replace old ones—is the only way forward emotionally. People with fibromyalgia need to look after their minds as well as their bodies.

If you have had to give up your job, studying part-time at your local college will help you feel less isolated. Whether you want to acquire a few academic qualifications or simply take up a new leisure interest—where the atmosphere is more casual and regular attendance not so important—learning something different can be rewarding. Studying a subject that is helpful in dealing with fibromyalgia—homeopathy, reflexology, aromatherapy, meditation, relaxation, stress management or assertiveness training, say—may prove invaluable, too.

Computer literacy and information technology courses can be useful if you are looking for a new career, want to a use a computer for your own purposes or are hoping to work from home. A college catalog can be obtained from your local library or the Internet. It is important that you inform your tutor of your fibromyalgia-related limitations at the outset.

Allowances will then be made if you are slow to produce work, time off will be understood and you may even be given the most comfortable chair!

If you are fairly mobile and employ caution, aqua-aerobics, low-impact aerobics or yoga classes can be beneficial. Such training should not only help maintain and ultimately improve your strength, stamina and mobility, it can also provide an outlet for stress. Competitive games— even those of a gentle nature such as chess, backgammon, roulette, bridge—are not a good idea. They produce tension and stress and, if you lose the game, feelings of uselessness and despair.

Perhaps you have already found that fibromyalgia itself can be the gateway to a whole new field of opportunity. Fibromyalgia support groups are springing up all over, each of which needs ongoing assistance of one kind or another. Practical help at group meetings and fundraising events is always required. If you are not physically able to tend an information booth or refreshment stand, you may be able to assist by contributing to the group's newsletter, donating sale goods or cookies for the next fundraiser, providing ideas for events or offering suggestions for speakers.

In fact, if you would like to involve yourself more in the group's activities, you could offer to become a committee member. People who participate in volunteer work invariably report a rise in their self-esteem. If your particular talent is handling money, you could offer to be treasurer; if you have clerical experience, you could volunteer to be secretary; if you are good at organizing or dealing with people, you could be social secretary, or if you enjoy writing, you could edit the newsletters. If you possess people skills, common sense and a management background (although this is not essential), maybe you could even think of setting up and chairing a support group of your own. There are still many areas without existing groups.

Smile for a while

"All things are cause either for laughter or weeping," wrote Roman philosopher Seneca. It is true that comedy and tragedy are close bedfellows, for both are reflex actions rooted in the central nervous system and its related hormones.

How we respond to a certain stimulus depends on our outlook on life. Letting go of the past and our fears for the future is "releasing." It allows us to smile more. The saying that "laughter is the best medicine" is particularly true for chronic pain patients. Laughter is also the most difficult emotional response to achieve when we are in pain. However, the people who manage to smile a lot, who manage to see the lighter side of different situations, deal more effectively with their pain. Fibromyalgia is not a funny condition—it causes a lot of grief and disability—yet a surprising number of sufferers retain (or evolve) a good sense of humor.

Laughing at yourself in particular can be more therapeutic than a whole-body massage, it can be more releasing than sex or alcohol, and it invariably makes other people warm to you. When you laugh, your muscles relax, bleak thoughts lift and "feel-good" endorphins are released into your bloodstream. As a result, you feel uplifted and bright!

Adjusting Your Lifestyle

On a more practical level, it is vital that people with fibromyalgia focus on all they do in the course of a day. Only by being constantly aware can you avoid unnecessary pain. Being conscious of the way you dress, sit and perform tasks requires a lot of effort, but can become second nature once you have learned to adjust behaviors identified as pain-provoking and reaped the benefits of doing this.

Identifying problems

As low muscle endurance causes numerous problems in fibromyalgia, try to always assess the possible repercussions before going ahead with any activity. Consider first the way you move. How do you get out of bed? Do you sit bolt upright, then climb clumsily out, or do you ease yourself to the edge, then carefully roll out? How do you shower? Do you scrub yourself vigorously or do you soap and sponge yourself carefully? How do you dress? Do you hop around on one leg as you struggle into your pantyhose or trousers, or do you sit down and carefully pull them on?

The operative word is "carefully." If you think yourself through your daily routine, you will likely find many examples of where the word "carefully" should be—but is not—applied. "Care" is perhaps your greatest weapon. Use it and you can prevent the muscle damage that leads to a full-scale flare-up, as well as the myriad of emotional problems tied into any exacerbation of symptoms.

Next, you should evaluate the way you perform tasks around the house. Housework has many pitfalls for fibromyalgics. Vacuuming is off limits for most sufferers, as are lifting furniture, decorating and heavy cleaning. Jobs such as cooking, baking, washing, ironing and shopping carry a high risk for some sufferers, and the possible repercussions should be considered carefully before going ahead.

If, for example, moving the sofa to clean behind it instigated a previous flare-up, ask yourself whether you really want a repeat performance. Try to learn from your experiences. Look for and examine possible solutions. Cooking, for instance, can be made easier by buying occasional microwave meals, frozen vegetables and takeout food. Show family members how grateful you are when they prepare a meal in advance and they may offer to do it regularly! However, lifting heavy pans from the cupboard and trays or dishes out of the oven is, for many fibromyalgics, too risky. The solution may be in timing the meal so that a family member can serve it on arriving home from work. If you are in no condition to even attempt cooking, you must find some way of passing the task to someone else. The key is to know your limitations and to abide by them.

Other housework—dusting, dishwashing, wiping kitchen surfaces, cleaning the bathroom and hanging out laundry—can seem too simple to even think of giving up. However, consider a moment the demands these activities exert on your energy-depleted, pain-disposed body. For a start, although dusting is viewed as a light task, it demands excesses of movement. You may need to kneel or bend to dust the hearth, you may need to stretch to dust the wall unit or bookshelves, you may need to lean over the TV to dust the window ledge. See what I mean? When you do the dishes, you stand still, often in a slightly hunched position, and scouring pans and baking trays requires you to exert a surprising amount of pressure. Wiping kitchen surfaces makes you tense, stoop and use pressure. Cleaning the bathroom requires that you bend, stretch and use pressure, and doing laundry involves bending, lifting and stretching!

All these movements can cause your pain levels to rise. If, after considering the possible consequences, you feel you can perform a task without there being a payback later, use caution anyway. Lifting anything moderately heavy is not wise. If you are fairly confident that you can lift, say, a wet sheet from the laundry basket, be sure that your back, hips and head are correctly aligned. When you need to use pressure, say when polishing or ironing, keep your body as relaxed as possible and take regular breaks. If you feel the slightest elevation of your normal levels of discomfort, rest immediately. There is always another day.

Re-evaluating non-essential activities

There are perhaps several activities that, although you know them to be risky, you nevertheless continue to perform. You would be well advised to regularly review their importance, however. For instance, you may unwittingly be aggravating your condition by washing your hair every morning in winter. If this is the case, ask yourself if it is crucial, now that temperatures have fallen and you're feeling delicate, that you do so. Wouldn't washing it once or twice a week be sufficient? Could you even consider having your hair restyled for the duration of winter? Easy-to-manage hairstyles are not necessarily unflattering!

Other "necessary" activities should be regularly assessed, too. For example, is it imperative that you dust the living room every day? Wouldn't once or twice a week be adequate here, too? Do underwear, dishtowels and so on desperately need ironing? Surely a few wrinkles in such items can be overlooked? Do you have to haul shopping all the way from the supermarket? Shopping is now available via the Internet or by phone to supermarkets that deliver the goods to your home at a time convenient to you. If such a service is not yet operating in your area, consider getting someone else to shop for you.

Depending on your present state of health, you could also ask yourself whether or not it is important that you do all the dishwashing. Wouldn't it be safer, if you are feeling fragile, to leave the dishes in water for someone else to deal with later? Do you have to go out to pay bills when you're really not up to it? Wouldn't it be easier to set up direct debits from your bank account? Should you really be trailing around town looking for household items when your legs are painful already? Wouldn't it be better to order them from a catalog?

Heeding past pain triggers

Fibromyalgia is a frustrating business, not least because the boundaries of what we can and cannot do are continually shifting. Delayed pain, arising from the low muscle stamina situation affecting all fibromyalgia sufferers, means that a task we accomplish with little payback one week can give rise to a full-scale flare-up the next. This factor is then complicated by a sensitivity to cold, heat, stress and so on. It is essential, therefore, that we learn from our experiences, taking account of all problem areas.

We are often at our lowest physical and emotional ebb during the early months/years of the illness, when, loath to abandon the activities that afford us a sense of self, purpose and worth, we are inclined to ignore past pain triggers. We are afraid of giving in to the illness, fearing that if we stop pushing ourselves, we may end up being incapable of anything. Only with the realization that such behavior is actually aggravating the illness do we eventually change our ways. Uncertainty regarding exactly where our boundaries lie, however, can cause us to then go through a period of overprotecting ourselves.

There is nothing more disconcerting than knowing that, in undertaking almost any activity, there is a risk of inducing an increase in pain or a full symptom flare-up. However, the risk can be minimized by constant wariness, remembering to always pace yourself, keeping your body relaxed and moving cautiously. Unfortunately, it is not possible to *eliminate* risk in fibromyalgia. Effectively coming to a full stop would arrest feelings of achievement, reduce stamina and cause muscle wastage. You can only retain, and ultimately improve, the strength you have by being as active as possible—without overdoing it! It is important that you constantly strive, therefore, to achieve a balance between too much and too little activity. "Easier said than done," I can almost hear you say and how right you are!

In order to achieve a balance—keeping in mind that the scales will keep tilting—you should consider past pain triggers. For example, if cleaning the car last month resulted in an exacerbation of pain, you should ask yourself these questions.

- Were you up to undertaking the task in the first place?
- Did you work just as quickly as before you got ill?

- Did you clean the whole car without pausing?
- Did you put on a spurt when your pain levels began rising?

A positive answer to any of the above would account for the extra pain! Now reassess the whole procedure. Wouldn't it, if you are well enough, be better to clean the interior on Monday morning, taking care to work slowly and carefully, then rest Monday afternoon? If there is no worsening of symptoms, maybe the windows could be cleaned on Tuesday and so on.

When, after due deliberation, you decide to tackle a certain task/activity, always attend to the way you go about it. Instead of preceding with the vigor born of long years of habit, take care to work slowly and cautiously, with your body in a stable and balanced position. It is equally important that you stop what you are doing and rest as soon as you feel your normal pain levels rising. If you don't break off immediately, you may bring on a flare-up lasting weeks!

Being assertive

Trying always to please others, put others first, is counterproductive. Rather than inspiring admiration, pushing yourself beyond your limits makes others suppose that you are doing what you are capable of doing. They will expect the same from you every time. Avoid risking extra pain and maintain your self-respect by learning to please yourself instead Try, too, to speak up when you need a helping hand.

Asking for help is not easy, especially when you have been active and independent all your life. Yet communicating your needs will usually get you what you want. What is the alternative? Frustration and anger. Asking for help is not an indication of weakness or failure. It is a sign of your resolve to face your situation, to be less of an emotional drain on the people around you. Rather than have you angry because they are unable to anticipate your needs, your partner or friend would surely prefer that you speak out.

There is a fine line between being assertive and being demanding, however! Asking for help clearly and politely, then showing gratitude afterwards creates "feel-good" emotions in others. It also increases the chances of their offering help in the future.

Encouraging flexibility in the people around you is important, too. It can reduce the pressure to "oblige." For example, preparing friends for a possible last-minute cancellation on your part minimizes their dis-appointment—and your resulting guilt—if you do have to cancel. Like-wise, warning co-workers that you may not be up to finishing that piece of work over the weekend prepares them for the possibility of having to do it on Monday.

Learning to say "no"

Saying "no" to others is equally difficult, but, for the sake of your health, you need to say it, and as often as necessary. Again, until told other-wise, the people in your life will simply assume you are still able to do most things.

If, after friends "expect" you to drive 20 miles to visit them, help them move furniture or babysit their toddler, your pleas of ill health are disregarded, your safest option is to say a definite "no." Go on to illus-trate exactly why you are refusing.

Taking the first example, you could explain, "If I drove over to you, I wouldn't be up to much else. It's been a while since we met, and I was looking forward to a good chat." Your friends will likely admit they didn't realize how ill you were and offer to drive to your home instead. However, if they are not satisfied with your reasoning, you should dig in your heels and add, "Then the drive home would be a nightmare. To be honest, I'd be in so much pain I wouldn't be safe behind the wheel! I'd be grateful if you could come to see me instead." If these people are worthy of the title "friends," they will now readily agree to your suggestion.

To the friends who expect you to help them move, you could say, "I'm sorry, but I can't. If I tried lifting furniture I'd end up rigid with pain—and I'm not exaggerating." If they have helped you a lot in the past, you could add, "I'll be happy to bring you a casserole, though." The response will probably be sympathy for your ill health, together with gratitude for offering alternative assistance.

To the friends who have asked you to babysit their toddler, you could say, "I'd love to look after little Katy, but I'm just not well enough. What most concerns me is that I wouldn't be able to leap up if she was about to hurt herself." Wanting the best for their daughter, your friends would probably say a hurried, "Oh, I see. Don't worry, we'll get so-and-so to look after her!"

Don't, in any circumstance, allow anyone to pressure you into doing something you know will provoke pain. Also, don't put yourself under pressure by feeling obliged to repay someone in kind. Your health is far more important than feelings of duty.

The People Around You

Fibromyalgics desperately need to know that others care. Most of all they crave the sympathy and understanding of their nearest and dearest, feeling upset when they are shown thoughtlessness or impatience. Yet sufferers often fail to appreciate that the illness can create huge problems for these very people.

Fibromyalgia and your partner

Our partners—on whom we tend to rely most for emotional support—are often more troubled by our ill health than we realize. They can feel guilty for being well and active when we are sick and stagnant, disappointed and confused when we show no sign of recovery, angry and useless for seeming never to be able to say the right thing and, not least, anxious for their own future happiness.

In fact, our partners' concerns are possibly equal to our own. Their need for intimacy, companionship and a future they can look forward to—mixed with feelings of inadequacy for being unable to ease our suffering—may even prompt doubts about their ability to cope indefinitely with a partner who is chronically ill. Their misgivings can then be amplified when they endure endless reproaches for being insensitive and uncaring.

A person who is chronically ill can become self-absorbed. The main causes are that:

- the physical and emotional drain of dealing with the condition can interfere with the sufferer's ability to see their partner's viewpoint; and
- after experiencing little but skepticism or indifference from others, the sufferer may misinterpret their partner's behavior as more of the same.

When a communication breakdown occurs, the relationship can become a battle, with each partner feeling resentful and unloved. Unless each makes an effort to understand the other person, the relationship may flounder. It is a fact that you can only know what your partner is thinking and feeling when you make time to calmly talk problems through. It is certainly worth the effort for exchanging perceptions, fears and needs carries the bonus of strengthening your relationship.

Fibromyalgia and other family members

Just as your partner has their own needs, so too have other family members. Their needs are essentially selfish, as are everyone's. In most cases, their chief need, where you are concerned, is to see you well and smiling again. They won't then have to worry about you so much, they won't then be obliged to be so attentive. Once you are "recovered," you will again be able to accompany them on Saturday shopping sessions, go to line dancing class, shoot pool and play tennis . . . . Put simply, you are an important part of their lives and they want everything to be back to normal.

As your illness continues, however, their bafflement may turn to irritation. Desperate to see you well, they may prefer to interpret your behavior as lethargy, self-indulgence or hypochondria rather than true chronic illness. Remarks such as, "You're not doing anything to help yourself," "You need to get out and enjoy yourself more" are typical, made in the misguided belief that you need a "push" to help you back to "normality."

Unchecked, such "advice" can turn to full-scale nagging. Comments such as, "You should try running up and down the stairs 20 times a day—that'll improve your stamina," "Get out on your bicycle again. It'll do you good," "Are you sure you're trying hard enough? Don't you want to get better?" may be delivered repeatedly in a genuine desire to see you fit and well, but, they are hurtful and demoralizing. When told often enough that you are making no effort to improve your condition, you can start to believe it.

Ironically, the people closest to us are the ones most likely to make damaging remarks, which fact only compounds our hurt. However, we should try to remember that they are the people who are most concerned that we get better. Instead of observing the situation from all angles, they make the mistake of seeing it through their eyes only.

DANIEL AND HELEN

It is easy to understand why 10-year-old Daniel has convinced himself that his mother, Helen, 39, is not as ill as she says she is. He needs her to make his meals, run him around in the car, organize his life . . . just to be there as her normal, capable self. He sees her illness as a threat to his whole world. She *looks* fine—just the same as ever. In attempting to prove to himself that everything is indeed exactly as it always was, Daniel will often say, "You look fine, Mom. Take me to my friend's house tonight, will you?" When Helen, feeling guilty, explains that she's not up to driving the car, Daniel bursts out, "You don't want to do anything for me any more! I don't think you love me!" So, despite the fact that Helen is in pain, she gets into the car and takes her son to see his friend. Consequently, Daniel is reassured, but Helen, in more pain than ever, is upset that her child can't seem to understand.

Daniel's demands persist because, in capitulating, Helen is proving she can still do as much as ever for him. He will only accept her illness if she continually reassures him of her love, yet firmly explains why she cannot be as active as before. When children know where they stand, they soon adapt.

SARAH AND MICHAEL

Sarah, 30, is mother to 18-month-old Bethany and has recently been diagnosed as having fibromyalgia. She makes keeping Bethany clean, safe and fed a priority, but feels a failure for neglecting the housework, annoyed that her husband, Michael, expects home life to be as happy and ordered as it was before she became ill and cheated for being too ill to enjoy Bethany.

Their respective parents occasionally offer to babysit, but Sarah invariably feels too ill to go out. This is yet another bone of contention between Michael and herself.

Fibromyalgics with young children need a lot of practical help and need to do a lot of straight talking to relatives and friends. Sarah cannot, realistically, be expected to care for a toddler all day, as well as perform all the other tasks in the home. She needs to calmly inform Michael, their families and close friends exactly how ill and miserable she feels, making it clear that, as well as daily help, she needs rest periods and quality time with her child. If no one volunteers assistance (people usually do offer to help at this point), she will need to ask for it outright. She and Michael should then ask family and friends to have Bethany on weekends—maybe draw up a rotation schedule.

PETER AND HIS PARENTS

Joan and Derek are parents of Peter, who is 48, married, and has two sons. Peter is a fibromyalgia sufferer. Joan and Derek have always enjoyed vacations with Peter and his family, but they now feel these are in jeopardy; they have proudly watched Peter's career, which he has suddenly abandoned and they had hoped to rely on him a bit more as they grew older. In addition, they formerly felt a sense of satisfaction at seeing him happy with his life. Observing that he is now unhappy and in pain has even induced feelings of failure in them. Many parents measure their parenting success by the health, happiness and prosperity of their children.

Finding it difficult to cope with Peter's anguish, unwilling to accept that he is as incapacitated as he says he is, they constantly compare "then" with "now." They see a man who has lost his "status" in life, whose wife and children are increasingly unhappy and, because he is no longer able to provide, is struggling financially. They make comparisons, with how active and alert they were at his age, how they enjoyed family life and how they managed to care for their own aging parents.

As Peter shows no signs of recovery, Joan and Derek's skepticism increases. They convince themselves that if he "pulls himself together" he will quickly return to normal. As more time elapses, they decide that his illness is imaginary, preferring to think he is suffering from mental instability than from fibromyalgia—a condition of which, after all, they have never heard.

Peter needs to sit down with his parents and firmly assert that their attitude is hurting him. Seen, for the first time, from their son's viewpoint, they will probably realize that their behavior has indeed been inappropriate and may even apologize. This is Peter's opportunity to tell them more about the illness, backing up his words with literature on the subject. His parents may occasionally revert to the old misconceptions but should be willing to re-evaluate their behavior as and when it is pointed out.

REBECCA AND HER MOTHER

Some family situations have become too fraught to simply be altered by a few firm words. Rebecca, 26, is resentful that 54-year-old Margaret, her fibromyalgic mother, is not there for her any more. She accuses Margaret of "wallowing in self-pity" and "demanding attention for an illness she hasn't got." Margaret reacts angrily and the situation quickly spirals out of control. Rebecca may even refuse to let her children see their grandmother, declaring that as she is "off her head," she would upset them. This state of events is profoundly disturbing to Margaret, for not only does she feel an incredible sense of loss (similar to that of being bereaved), she may also assume she is responsible for the rift.

Rather than trying to get through to her daughter, Margaret would be best advised to keep out of her life for a time. However, she must remember that she has done nothing wrong. She suffers from a debilitating illness, which should be received with an open mind. Okay, so she lost her temper when Rebecca was mean, but that is understandable. In waiting for Rebecca to calm down, she offers her daughter an opportunity to examine *her* behavior.

If some times elapses and still Rebecca makes no contact, I would suggest that Margaret make the first move. She should say, "I'm sorry things got so heated. I said some stupid things." I anticipate that Rebecca will also apologize, allowing her mother to add, "I have been very ill, and I get frustrated when you don't seem to understand. Can we talk about it some more?" If Rebecca again erects a brick wall, it is best to keep some distance between them. However, I expect that, at this juncture, Rebecca will make more of an effort to understand.

Coping with Chronic Pain

Pain is transmitted to the brain via two types of nerves, each working independently of the other and each having a different structure. "Fast pain"—that arising from a cut, toothache, or broken limb—is quickly relayed to the central nervous system (CNS) located in the brain, but the actual pain is felt at the level of the tissues, often provoking a reflex action of instantly withdrawing from the pain source. In fast pain, the hurt can stop fairly rapidly, too.

"Deep pain," on the other hand, travels relatively slowly, and the resulting pain sensations are felt at the level of the CNS. This type of pain lingers longer than that of fast pain, its transmissions normally associated with chronic pain conditions such as fibromyalgia, rheumatoid arthritis and osteoarthritis. The "spillover" of certain chemicals in the muscles in fibromyalgia further aggravates the situation, causing the sensation of pain to spread to nearby healthy tissues—in this instance perhaps traveling from the neck into the shoulders, back, face and jaw.

Although a small proportion of the pain of fibromyalgia is thought to be fast pain—felt at tissue level—the greater proportion is believed to be deep pain. Individuals with a deep pain problem are also far less likely to obtain relief from painkilling medication, (narcotics and analgesics) than do those with a fast-pain problem. However, new kinds of medication continue to emerge, and medical professionals are becoming more open to using "invasive" treatments for severe pain.

Natural painkillers

On a more positive note, we also know that the body is capable of generating painkilling "feel-good" neurotransmitters (endorphins and enkephalins) by natural means. Pleasurable activities, positive thinking, total relaxation and exercise (careful, non-taxing exercise where fibromyalgia is concerned) can all produce a satisfying "high" or feelings of serenity. Both states actively block a degree of pain. Alternatively, negative thoughts and feelings, along with long-term inactivity and/or dependency on medication, can suppress the production of these "feel-good" chemicals, thereby limiting the individual's ability to deal with pain.

Distraction

Living with chronic pain is a formidable affair. The awareness that we may never be entirely rid of it creates negative emotions that, if we fail to devise ways of managing the pain, can be overwhelming.

The simplest coping strategy is distraction. Awareness of pain fades when the mind is pleasantly occupied. The intensity of any pain, however, can be greatly influenced by the situation in which it is experienced. Throughout history, there have been numerous accounts of soldiers fighting on despite terrible injuries, only becoming conscious of their pain when the battle was over. The theory that circumstances peculiar to each case are responsible for a variance in pain levels was supported by research in the 1950s, when it was found that wounded soldiers complained far less during recuperation than did civilians facing various types of surgery. The main difference was that the former had many distractions from their pain. They felt relief at still being alive and knew that, for them, the battle was over and they would likely soon be returned to their families, all of which probably acted as a painkiller in itself. The civilians, on the other hand, had no such strong positive thoughts about their stay in hospital. Indeed, they were worried about spending time in alien surroundings, being away from their families and, not least, about the operation going wrong.

The distraction technique can easily be applied to our everyday lives. For example, engaging in cheery conversation, reading a lighthearted book, watching a comedy on TV, lovemaking or experiencing pleasing therapies such as aromatherapy or reflexology can occupy the senses and effectively reduce the awareness of pain. Indeed, finding pleasurable distractions can be one of our greatest allies in our quest to manage the pain.

However, beware! Due to the delayed response situation caused by low muscle endurance—the presence of which typifies fibromyalgia—pain must never be entirely blocked from the conscious mind. Anticipation is your best weapon here. In the early stages of pain progression, stop and think what you need to do in order to intercept its course. In order to detect an early build up of pain, constant, low-key awareness of your body is essential.

Staying active

When you feel constantly wiped out, when it seems that all you do causes pain, it may be tempting to take to your bed. Limited bed-rest is beneficial in a flare-up, but if you don't attempt to exercise your body on a fairly regular basis, your body can become stiff and less efficient and your limbs more painful. and your muscles will likely waste.

Holding yourself stiffly encourages pain, as does limiting yourself from making specific movements. If, for example, your neck is painful when you move your head, trying to avoid doing so indefinitely will cause the muscles to become less flexible and enforced movement to become more painful. It's a Catch-22 situation. You limit your head movements because they cause pain, then, because your neck muscles become weaker, the pain increases. The only answer—painful though it may be—is to begin gentle neck exercises.

Crisis medication

We live in a society that is overly reliant on drugs. A prescription for medication of some kind is expected of a visit to the doctor, and self-medication is encouraged by media advertising. Painkillers, anti-inflammatory drugs and muscle relaxants are beneficial in the short term, but prolonged usage can produce side effects ranging from mild digestive problems to liver or kidney damage, as well as tolerance, which is when the patient needs to take more and more of a certain drug to achieve the same effect. Another side effect may be "brain fog," which impedes the clear thinking often required to regain control over your life.

Medication can, however, reduce pain to a level at which gentle exercise can be resumed, thereby strengthening the tissues. In the early stages of illness, it can also help to reduce underlying tension. These benefits aside, because, with time, their side effects often surpass their benefits, they are best used briefly. Long-term pain management can, be more successfully achieved by natural means.

Electrical stimulators

Transcutaneous electrical nerve stimulator (TENS) machines provide effective pain relief for many people, without the risk of side effects. The small, battery operated devices, easily attached to the waist-band of a skirt or trousers, transmit electrical impulses to electrodes that adhere to painful areas. The machine produces a tingling/pulsating sensation as it transmits electrical impulses to the CNS, thereby blocking sensations of pain.

In addition, electrical stimulation is believed to encourage the release of endorphins—the natural painkillers produced in the brain. TENS machines can be worn from early morning until bedtime, but up to one hour of usage may be required before benefit is felt.

The people who are lucky enough to experience relief using their TENS machines daily may be able to eliminate drugs entirely. However, many find that, although the treatment works well at first, it becomes less effective after a few weeks. This probably occurs because the CNS overrides the effects of repeated interference. Devices that overcome this problem by randomly switching stimulation on and off are currently being developed. In the meantime, using the machine for maybe two hours, then turning it off for two hours (or whatever timescale is relevant to your levels of pain) can prolong its usefulness.

Improving sleep

Pain levels commonly rise when sleep is more disturbed than usual. Stress is often at the root of sleep disturbance, for there is nothing worse for mind and body than anxiously tossing and turning. When stress can be relieved by a simple positive action, however, do it! For example, explaining to a friend that you aren't up to a particular activity or securing a promise of help with your weekend shopping should immediately put your mind at ease.

When stress arises due to a deep-seated concern—maybe you are worried that, because you are stumbling over your words more lately, your condition is deteriorating, or perhaps you know your son is playing hooky from school—the problem should be resolved as soon as possible. In the first instance, you should see your doctor at your earliest opportunity. Hopefully, the doctor will quickly reassure you that a good relaxation strategy will effectively restore—or at least improve—your speech. (If you ask for details in this respect, the doctor will point you in the right direction.) In the second instance, you and your partner should talk with the child in order to discover the root of the problem. You should then devise with his teachers a stage-1 rescue plan. With any luck, you will soon be sleeping better.

Over-the-counter medications can increase the duration of sleep, but will not lengthen deep sleep, essential for the repair and regeneration of tissues. Tricyclic antidepressants, available on prescription, can encourage deep sleep. If your prescribed medication is no longer effective, the dosage may need adjusting.

When pain prevents you from getting to sleep, try taking your usual painkillers at bedtime. If discomfort due to lying in one position for too long wakes you up, evaluate the comfort of your bed. Although a reasonably firm bed is recommended for fibromyalgics, you may find it helps to place a duvet between the mattress and sheet. The surface "give" this offers is kind on sore muscles. Neck support in the form of a surgical collar or a specially molded pillow can be helpful, too. When lying on your back, place a pillow beneath your knees to take the strain off your lower back, hips and legs.

Develop good sleep habits by doing the following:

- unwind before going to bed by listening to music or a relaxation tape, reading or watching an unemotive program on TV;
- have a warm drink;
- shortly before bedtime, take a warm bath (preferably using relaxing aromatherapy oils);
- go to bed as soon as you feel sleepy—don't wait up until your usual bedtime;
- ensure that your bed and bedroom are warm;
- once in bed, breathe slowly and evenly, not shallowly, but using your diaphragm (page 132), clear your mind and allow your thoughts to drift—don't hold on to any one thought, let each pass unchecked;
- get up at the same time every morning.

Try to avoid the following:

- caffeine drinks after 6 p.m.;
- engaging in animated conversation or arguments before bedtime;
- napping during the day;
- sitting watching TV for long periods, particularly in the evening.

Taking up the last point, sitting to watch TV for several hours during the daytime and evening is, for many of us, a habit that not only causes stiffness—and, therefore, added pain—but also interferes with sleep. TV provokes numerous emotional responses in rapid succession. It quickens the heart rate and releases chemicals (such as adrenaline) for no useful purpose. When these chemicals are produced naturally, we deal with the situation and blood flow is returned to normal. However, when chemicals are induced second-hand, by watching TV, they remain in the bloodstream. This causes tension to linger and, ultimately, gives rise to more pain.

Keeping warm

As we well know, cold has an adverse effect on fibromyalgics. Sitting in a draft can cause our muscles to stiffen and our pain levels to rise, and standing at a bus stop in a bitterly cold wind can provoke a severe flare-up. Although we don't always do what is best for us, we soon learn to avoid such situations. When we take steps to keep warm at all times, wrapping up when we go outside and making sure we stay warm indoors too, muscle flexibility is encouraged.

Direct application of heat usually releases muscle tension. It increases blood flow through the tissues, encouraging oxygenation and removing toxins. Direct heat can come in the form of warm showers or baths, infrared heat lamps, microwavable wheat bags, electric under and over blankets, hot water bottles, electric heating pads and muscle-warming massage cream.

The use of cold

Trigger points or other painful areas are often more responsive to the application of cold than they are to heat. Placed directly over a painful area, an ice pack, for example, can moderate the transmission of pain messages to the CNS. (An ice pack, bag of frozen peas or refrigerator-cooled wheat bag, should never be placed directly on the skin but wrapped in a dish towel.) A routine of 10 minutes on, then 10 minutes off is recommended.

Relaxing the muscles

When we are anxious or in pain, we subconsciously tighten our muscles, which causes more pain. It is important, therefore, that people with fibromyalgia learn to recognize increasing tenseness and make efforts to check involuntary tightening.

The technique of tightening and then relaxing different muscle groups is not recommended in fibromyalgia. The mere act of tightening can give rise to pain that is not easy to shift.

Action for flare-ups

Flare-ups of pain are an ever-present risk in fibromyalgia. They can be caused by:

- the physical stress of repetitive work;
- emotional stress and/or insomnia;
- a fall or bump;
- cold or damp weather conditions;
- hormonal changes brought about by the menstrual cycle.

When a sufferer makes no attempt to manage the pain of a flare-up, their condition may rapidly deteriorate. This can create feelings of anger and despair, which, in turn, increases pain. Unless the following factors are carefully observed, the situation can become very difficult.

Self-help plan for flare-ups

1. Recognize when your pain levels are rising. Take action before it gets worse. This may include immediate rest, application of heat or cold, painkilling or muscle-relaxing medication, massage, myofascial (trigger point) release therapy, aromatherapy treatment, relaxation and meditation exercises, use of a TENS machine or whatever works best for you.

2. Be positive! A positive frame of mind speeds recovery. Tell yourself, "I'll get through this just as I have before," "I am more aware of how to help myself this time," "I'll make efforts to distract myself," "I won't let myself get depressed. I know that does more harm than good."

3. Explore the possible reasons for the increase in pain. Ask yourself, "Did I overexert myself?" "Did I forget to pace myself?" "Should I have driven the car when I was already feeling fragile?" "Did I sit in one position for too long?" "Was I leaning forward too much?"

4. Decide how you can reduce the risk of future flare-ups. Do this by asking for help when you need it, being clearer about what you can and can't do and aligning your expectations of yourself and others with what is practicable. All of these are helpful emotionally as well as physically.

5. Review the effectiveness of your current flare-up strategy. Is your present medication adequate in a crisis? Can you do anything fur-

ther to help you stay positive? Is it time to visit your doctor again? Could you try a new type of complementary therapy?

Stress Management

Stress arises not only as a result of what happens to us, but also from our reactions to these things. Negative attitudes can actually cause people to see catastrophe in what to others would be normal, everyday events. When a situation is interpreted as a crisis, adrenaline is released into the bloodstream and the body automatically puts itself "on alert." Breathing becomes shallow and fast, the heart rate quickens, blood pressure rises and the muscles tense, allowing the individual to deal with an emergency more effectively. These responses can be destructive, however, when they occur frequently.

Delay your reaction

Because living with a chronic pain condition naturally creates stress in daily life, fibromyalgics experience higher levels of stress than do non-sufferers. However, curbing your responses to certain occurrences can greatly reduce stress buildup and the incidence of flare-ups. As a troublesome event unfolds, try not to react instantly. By postponing your response, you allow yourself time to evaluate the situation, to see it as it really is. Now select a response that doesn't create more stress.

Self-talk

The way we speak to ourselves has great bearing on our stress levels. When we analyze our thoughts, we are often surprised at their negativity, but they must be examined before we can begin to change their destructive pattern. When the TV breaks down, for example, your first thoughts may be, "It's so unfair! I was really looking forward to watching that film," "This is all I need! I can't afford a new TV," "Even if it can be repaired, it will probably cost a small fortune" "What am I supposed to do with my time—sit twiddling my thumbs?"—stress-provoking thoughts by any standard!

By being aware that negative thoughts create stress, you can train yourself into more positive self-talk. Using the same example, you may instead think, "I'll call around for quotes in the morning. Maybe it won't cost much to repair," "It was on its last legs anyway. I'll take the opportunity to buy a more up-to-date TV," "I could buy a new TV on a 0 percent lease-purchase deal," "I could buy a reconditioned TV if I can't afford a new one," "I could rent one and not have to worry about repair costs," "I wonder if my friend down the road is watching that film" or "In the meantime, this is my chance to read that book, finish my tapestry, phone Aunt Betty . . . ."

The following examples of stress-relieving self-talk can be applied to many potentially stressful situations.

"I'll break this problem into separate sections. They'll be easier to handle."

"I'll take things one step at a time."

"Is this really worth getting upset and angry over?"

"I've coped before, so I'll cope again."

"I can always ask for help if I need it."

"It could have been much worse."

"This is hardly a matter of life or death!"

"There's nothing I can do about this situation, so I will have to accept it."

Life stress evaluation

If you take time to evaluate all the relationships and activities in your everyday life, you are likely to find that some prompt more stress than benefit. Fibromyalgia demands that you protect your body and nourish your mind. "Involvements" that have ceased to do this are probably harmful.

In reviewing your relationships and activities, however, remember that personal interactions and energy-related performances will always produce a certain amount of stress. It is when the stress outweighs the positive gains that you need to consider limiting or ceasing your involvement in them.

Address your stress

- List aspects of looking after the home that cause stress. Taking each problem in turn, can you make things easier for yourself? For example, you could try asking for help, sharing the housework, or accepting that you will have an untidier house in future.

- *List the stressful aspects of your job.* How can you make these things less stressful? For example, you could inform your boss and co-workers of your limitations, not place yourself under pressure, reduce your hours, find less taxing employment.
- *List personal relationships that are particularly stressful.* Taking each in turn, how exactly can you improve the situation? For example, could you express your needs and feelings more clearly, lower your expectations of the person(s) in question, limit your interactions with such people?
- *List the organizations, societies or groups that create more stress than benefit.* Remember that partaking in group activities can be diverting, uplifting and give you a real sense of purpose. Try to be honest about whether the stress really does outweigh the gains. If there is truly a problem, how exactly can you improve the situation? Perhaps you could inform the person in charge that you need to limit your duties, take on a different and perhaps more rewarding role, take a break from your involvement for a period or even end your association with the organization.

Chronic Stress

Chronic stress is the state of being constantly "on alert." The physiological changes associated with this state—a fast heart rate, shallow breathing and muscle tension—persist over a long period, making relaxation difficult. Chronic stress can lead to nervousness, hypertension, irritability and depression.

The condition commonly arises when any of the following needs fail to be met on a long-term basis.

• *The need to be understood*
Although this subject has been discussed earlier in this chapter, I will reiterate that people with fibromyalgia long to talk truthfully about how they feel and be taken at their word. Being misunderstood can induce frustration, irritability and despondency. Feelings of helplessness (you cannot change other people's minds) and isolation (you learn

not to expect to be understood) may arise too, causing you to shut others out. However, it is not easy for others to accept and understand, particularly when your illness affects their needs. Sharing your feelings without blaming anyone is the most important step toward being understood.

• *The need to be loved*
Feeling unlovable is doubtless the greatest threat to the emotional well-being of fibromyalgics. You may tell yourself you have more to worry about than your appearance, yet feel concern that your partner now finds you unattractive and so will ultimately end the relationship, and this may make you subconsciously withdraw your affections. You may wonder how anyone *could* love you the way you are looking, for you may have developed "pain lines" around your eyes and mouth, you may have dark shadows beneath your eyes and, due to inactivity, you may have put on weight. You may even have become miserable, irrational and antagonistic. Moreover, you doubt anyone could really love a chronic pain sufferer, who would severely limit their life.

Before you can be loved by others, you need to love yourself. You need to see yourself as a worthwhile person with qualities that you, as well as others, can respect. Don't let apathy rule. Start the way you mean to go on by doing the following:

- make a list of your 10 best attributes;
- do one nice thing (however small) for another person each day, and don't forget to congratulate yourself for doing it;
- make the most of your appearance, within your physical and financial scope;
- regularly treat yourself to something uplifting—an aromatherapy or reflexology massage, for example;
- try to frequently indulge in something that stimulates your mind as well as creating a sense of fulfillment.

• *The need to love*
Fibromyalgia can cause introversion. It can cause you to wholly focus on your symptoms, ultimately withdrawing from those around you. However, loving others and actively attempting to cheer them can have a positive impact on your own life. For example, encouraging your

partner to smile can lift your own mood, phoning a friend with relationship problems can make you feel useful and having a nice chat with a lonely neighbor can hearten you both.

Where pleasing others is concerned, a careful balance must be sought, though. Fibromyalgics are often inclined to put others first. Saying "yes" to a request to pick up young Rosie from school because her mom is doing some decorating can be counterproductive if you are having a bad day yourself. Besides being angry with yourself for overdoing it, you may feel used. Rosie's mom is more able than you. She could have picked the child up herself.

In giving to others, you must be careful not to exceed your limitations. You can make someone smile with a few carefully chosen words, and a bit of honest flattery will make you feel just as good as the recipient. Instead of being defensive around others, try to understand their needs. They will likely be pleased and uplifted by the effort you have made and, hopefully, will want to respond in kind. You have to give before you can hope to receive.

• *The need to achieve*
Although the subject of "achievement" has been discussed earlier in this chapter, I will just add here that, in general, we are happy when we are producing something, when we feel we are of value. To be unproductive creates boredom and restlessness and giving up fulfilling activities breeds doubts about ever again experiencing feelings of achievement. However, those feelings really can be regained when, in accepting our limits, we carefully pace activities we previously enjoyed or take up rewarding substitute activities.

• *The need to be supported*
Fibromyalgics need the emotional and physical backing of others. Asking for help can feel humiliating, especially when we are used to priding ourselves on our capabilities. When we refuse to request assistance, however, we can get upset about others failing to second-guess our needs and we fret about the effects of doing too much ourselves. In order to avoid these negative emotions, do ask and try not to make the mistake of being unappreciative when others lend a hand. Accept help with good grace and your stress levels will automatically drop.

• *The need to be yourself*
The roles many of us play out, perhaps unaware, often have their origins in early childhood. If, for example, the parents of young Carl were scathing of incompetence when he was growing up, he may prize competence himself into adulthood, going so far as to hide instances when he is less than perfect. Only when he moves in with a partner who is far from perfect, a partner who is maybe even intimidated by Carl's apparent "perfection," will he begin to see that it is all right to be flawed.

There may be several ways in which you hide your real self. You may, for example, have been out with a person who lived and breathed football. You liked him a lot so you read the sports pages and feigned interest. However, realistically, going through life pretending to be interested in something you don't actually care a lot about causes untold stress. It is far better to be yourself for, apart from minimizing stress, you also know that the people important to you like you for who you really are.

• *The need to feel well*
Constantly feeling unwell is perhaps the most forbidding aspect of fibromyalgia. However, as we find our feet, we can take steps to lessen our awareness of illness as well as the severity of the condition itself. For instance, we can eat healthily, take regular (careful) exercise, avoid the foods and other substances to which we know we are sensitive, forge satisfactory relationships with our doctors, families and friends, learn the art of positive thinking and try different complementary therapies. Whether or not the benefits are only temporary, the feeling that we are actively helping ourselves creates a sense of achievement. In addition, activities that challenge the mind can help reduce feelings of uselessness and are fundamental to building self-esteem. They also lower stress levels.

When essential needs are not met

For fibromyalgics, meeting these seven essential needs is far from easy. Sufferers may be neither understood, nor supported, so they feel unlovable, fear they have little to offer others, feel devalued, limit their achievements they rarely feel well. Against such odds, the road ahead is undeniably bumpy. However, knowing your emotional needs—and endeavoring to meet them—will undoubtedly have a positive effect on your pain and stress levels.

Relaxation Techniques

Fibromyalgia is a condition for which, at present, medical science can do very little. Although experts by no means advocate that we should "grin and bear" the pain, it is advisable that fibromyalgia-related medication be used as sparingly as possible, given individual circumstances. Fibromyalgics achieve most success by means of self-help, many forms of which have been outlined earlier. However, the purest forms of self-help are deep breathing, relaxation and meditation—all natural therapies you can do yourself.

Deep breathing

In normal breathing, we take oxygen from the atmosphere down into our lungs. The diaphragm contracts, and air is pulled into the chest cavity. When we breath out, we expel carbon dioxide and other waste gases back into the atmosphere. However, when we are stressed or upset, or just from habit, we tend to use the rib muscles to expand the chest, breathing more quickly, sucking in air and breathing it out shallowly. This is good in a crisis as it allows us to obtain the optimum amount of oxygen in the shortest possible time, providing our bodies with the extra power needed to handle the emergency.

Some people do tend to get stuck in shallow, chest-breathing mode. In the long term, shallow breathing is not only detrimental to our physical and emotional health, it can also lead to hyperventilation, panic attacks, chest pains, dizziness and gastrointestinal problems.

To test your breathing, ask yourself the following questions.

- How fast are you breathing as you are reading this?
- Are you pausing between breaths?
- Are you breathing with your chest or with your diaphragm?

A DEEP BREATHING EXERCISE

The following deep breathing exercise should, ideally, be performed daily.

1. Make yourself comfortable, lying down in a warm room where you know you will be undisturbed for at least half an hour.
2. Close your eyes and try to relax.
3. Gradually slow down your breathing, inhaling and exhaling as evenly as possible.

4. Place one hand on your chest and the other on your abdomen, just below your ribcage.
5. As you inhale steadily and slowly through your nose, allow your abdomen to swell upward. Your chest should barely move.
6. As you exhale steadily and slowly through your mouth, let your abdomen flatten. Empty your lungs completely.

Give yourself a few minutes to get into a smooth, easy rhythm. As worries and distractions arise, don't hang onto them—wait calmly for them to float out of your mind, then focus once more on your breathing.

When you feel ready to end the exercise, open your eyes. Allow yourself time to become alert before rolling over on to one side and getting up. With practice, you will start to breathe with your diaphragm quite naturally all the time, and in times of stress you should be able to correct your breathing without too much effort.

Deep relaxation

Relaxation is one of the forgotten skills in today's hectic world. We already know that stress—which can give rise to muscle tension, insomnia, hypertension and depression—is perhaps the greatest enemy of the fibromyalgia sufferer. It is advisable, therefore, to learn at least one relaxation technique. The following exercise is perhaps the easiest.

A DEEP RELAXATION EXERCISE

1. Make yourself comfortable in a place where you will not be disturbed. Listening to restful music may help you relax.
2. Begin to slow down your breathing, inhaling steadily and slowly through your nose for a count of two, ensuring that the abdomen pushes outward as you breathe in.
3. Now exhale slowly and steadily through your mouth for a count of four, five or six.
4. After a couple of minutes, concentrate on each part of the body in turn, starting with your right arm. Consciously relax each set of muscles, allowing the tension to flow right out. Let your arm feel heavier and heavier as every last remnant of tension seeps away. Follow this procedure with the muscles of your left arm, then the muscles of your face, neck, stomach, hips and, finally, your legs and feet.

Visualization

When you have reached Step 4 of the deep relaxation exercise above, visualization can be introduced. As you continue to breathe slowly and evenly, imagine yourself surrounded, perhaps, by lush, peaceful countryside, beside a gently trickling stream or maybe on a deserted tropical beach, beneath swaying palm fronds, listening to the sounds of the ocean, thousands of miles from your worries and cares. Let the warm sun, the gentle breeze, the peacefulness of it all wash over you.

The tranquility you feel at this stage can be enhanced by frequently repeating the exercise—once or twice a day is best. With time, you should be able to switch into a calm state of mind whenever you feel stressed.

I will reiterate that relaxed muscles use far less energy than tense ones and that improved breathing leads to better circulation and oxygenation, which, in turn, helps the muscles and connective tissues. A relaxed mind can also greatly aid concentration and short-term memory. It can help eliminate "brain fog," too. All positive benefits, I'm sure you'll agree!

Meditation

Arguably the oldest natural therapy, meditation is the simplest and most effective form of self-help. Ideally, you should initially be taught the technique by a teacher, but, as meditation is essentially performed alone, it can be learned alone with equal success.

The unusual thing about meditation is that it involves "letting go," allowing the mind to roam freely. However, as most of us are used to striving to control our thoughts, letting go is not so easy as it sounds.

It may help to know that people who regularly meditate say they have more energy, require less sleep, are less anxious and feel far "more alive" than before they did so. Studies have shown that, during meditation, the heartbeat slows, blood pressure lowers and circulation improves, making the hands and feet feel much warmer.

Meditation may, to some people, sound a bit offbeat, something hippies do, but isn't it worth a try—especially when you can do it for free? Kick off those shoes and make yourself comfortable, somewhere you can be undisturbed for a while. Now follow these simple instructions.

First steps in meditation

1. Close your eyes, relax and practice the deep breathing exercise described above.

2. Concentrate on your breathing. Try to free your mind of conscious control. Letting it roam unchecked, try to allow the deeper, more serene part of you to take over.

3. If you wish to go farther into meditation, concentrate now on mentally repeating a "mantra"—a certain word or phrase. It should be something positive, such as "relax," "I feel calm," "I am feeling much better" or "I am special," whatever works best for you.

4. When you are ready to finish, open your eyes and allow yourself time to adjust to the outside world before getting to your feet.

The aim of repeating a mantra, mentally or actually out loud, is to plant the positive thought into your subconscious mind. It is a form of self-hypnosis, and only you control the messages placed there.

PART II

The Fibromyalgia Healing Diet

7

Basic Considerations for Health

Hunger is the body's alarm system telling us to eat. When our blood sugar levels are low, the body sends out this alarm, telling us to eat sugars, and when the body needs more liquid, it sends out an alarm telling us to drink. However, few people recognize that the body sends out these messages when a diet is lacking something it needs. These alarms come in the form of lethargy, sleeplessness, low mood, miscellaneous aches and pains and, eventually, chronic disease. It makes sense, then, to say that healing can best come from improvements in nutrition.

You may be surprised to hear that food is one of the finest medicines we can put into our bodies, one of the best means of influencing our health, but it is true. Not only does food keep us alive, it also has the ability to repair and regenerate our body's tissues.

Unfortunately, our diets have become very poor over the years. Nowadays, because of chemical pesticides, food additives, preservatives and so on, we constantly ingest low levels of toxins, which has given rise to an array of immune disorders. Fibromyalgia is one such disorder.

Why Good Nutrition?

The human body possesses all the necessary systems for regeneration, rejuvenation and repair. When provided with the right conditions, mentally and physically, the body will quite often heal itself, working at optimum efficiency and staving off disease. The most important factor influencing good physical health is good nutrition. It allows our cells—the smallest but most important components in our bodies—to be nourished continually and washed clean of waste. The cells will not function efficiently if they are seldom fed and cleansed.

Poor nutrition, on the other hand, causes a gradual toxic buildup within the cells. It can even lead to cell death. Junk food is a fine example of poor nutrition, for not only does it carry few nutrients, its digestion and detoxification draws energy from the body that could otherwise be used in thinking, working, playing and so on. In addition, poor-quality foods are difficult for the body to eliminate. As a result, bowel movements become irregular and toxic substances are absorbed into the body.

Many experts believe that fibromyalgia may arise as a result of toxic overload. When the liver—our main detoxification organ—is unable to keep up with the removal of toxins, they are deposited in the muscle fibers and connective tissues, causing pain and discomfort.

It is vital that people with fibromyalgia eat the right foods. Disease occurs when the body is vulnerable, when it is run down and crying out for help, as shown by fatigue, anxiety, insomnia, low mood and so on. However, when the cause of the problem is being treated, rather than the effect—as is the case when a nutritious diet is being followed—healing is likely to take place.

In fibromyalgia, there are abnormalities in the immune system (antibody protection against disease), the endocrine system (hormone levels) and the central nervous system (the body's nerve signaling system located in the brain and spinal cord). This section of the book is dedicated to suggesting the foods and nutritional supplements you can use to help return these systems to normal.

The Way We Were

Our bodies, physiologically speaking, have barely changed since the Stone Age. Available foodstuffs remain largely unchanged, too. What has changed, and in a relatively short period of time, is our diet and behavior. We now eat a wide variety of "processed" foods—that is, foods grown using chemicals and preservatives, flavorings, colorings and so on added before we eat them—in a stressful environment.

Stone Age people, on the other hand, had all the time in the world, except when under direct threat. Their foods were not sprayed with chemicals or injected with preservatives, they were eaten fresh and in season—and fresh, uncontaminated fruit and vegetables are highly nutritious. They are also rich in enzymes—the substances that aid digestion. For the most part, the food was uncooked, too. Unfortunately, cooking above 107°F and refrigeration both destroy the live digestive enzymes that help our bodies to break down food.

Stone Age people would also have eaten one type of food at a time. For example, when blackberries came into season, they would make whole meals of this fruit. This is quite unlike what we do today, when we combine several types of food at one sitting. It is a sad fact that we generally place more importance on taste than quality.

Fed on freshly gathered, uncontaminated foods, the digestive systems of Stone Age people would have functioned superbly, and the added benefit of fresh air and exercise contributed to their good health. It is doubtful that Stone Age people developed fibromyalgia. This disorder has seemingly become prevalent only in the last 100 years and, unfortunately, its incidence is rising all the time.

Foodstuffs Today

Since our Stone Age ancestors' time, we have developed the following habits so that, today:

- we eat food grown on artificially fertilized land and sprayed several times with chemical pesticides, which kill essential soil microbes that would otherwise help plants to absorb the nutrient-rich minerals essential to good health;
- plant foods are then artificially ripened, stored and processed;
- we generally prefer taste to quality;
- we eat foods out of season because they are readily available;
- we eat the tasty parts of the food only, disposing of the rest—for example, wheat husks are removed before the remaining cereal is processed into white flour—but "whole" foods aid the removal of waste materials from the bowel, so are vital to good bowel health;
- we eat hurriedly, often while working or thinking about problems;
- we dilute the nutrients in our food by drinking at the same time.

Recommendations for Fibromyalgia

In order to begin healing itself, the body requires a wide variety of foods and food combinations. To eat the same foods repeatedly means missing out on many important building blocks of life, for certain foods build and regenerate only certain parts of the body. A restricted diet also increases the risk of developing immune system disorders such as fibromyalgia.

Because the majority of our foodstuffs are grown in a chemical environment, they are low in nutrients and high in toxicity. It is advisable, therefore, to purchase organically grown produce and look for foods that are without added chemicals (colorings, flavorings, preservatives and so on).

Essential guidelines for achieving healing from fibromyalgia are as follows.

- Eat three or four small meals a day, with snacks in between.
- Never go more than two to three hours without eating, which means you should never go hungry.
- Do not skip breakfast. After fasting during the night, the body needs glucose. When nourishment is withheld, brain function is diminished. Studies have shown that children who eat breakfast perform better at school than those who have not eaten.
- Avoid missing a meal. When we allow ourselves to become very hungry, the sugary, high-fat foods that are bad for us become more tempting.
- Ensure your snacks are nutritious and readily available. Good examples are raw fruits and vegetables, fruit and vegetable juices, dried fruit, unsalted uncoated nuts (unless you have a nut allergy, of course), a variety of seeds and rye crispbreads. These should not spoil your appetite for an upcoming meal. At least half of your calorie intake should be made up of complex carbohydrates. These include fruits, vegetables and whole grains, such as bulgar wheat, couscous, millet, barley, brown rice and whole wheat.
- Fats (oils) should comprise approximately 20 to 25 percent of your calorie intake. *Unsaturated* fats (also known as polyunsaturated fats) are greatly beneficial to health. These include olive, safflower, sunflower and corn oils. *Saturated* fats, however, are

largely derived from animals and should be consumed in moderation, if at all. Examples are lard, butter and meat drippings.

- Protein should make up approximately 20–25 percent of your total calorie intake. Sources include chicken, turkey, fish (including tuna and salmon), beans, legumes (peas, beans and peanuts). Red meat is considered by some experts to be detrimental to fibromyalgics. However, my opinion is that small cuts of lean red meat, eaten only once or twice a week, are harmless. Meat is also one of the few sources of vitamin B_{12}.
- Eat plenty of fiber in the form of fruits, vegetables, whole-grain breads, cereals and legumes.
- Minimize your intake of sugar. Use raw honey, date sugar, molasses, barley malt and so on in place of table sugar and artificial sweeteners such as aspartame and saccharin.
- Junk foods and fast foods are loaded with harmful additives. Avoid them if at all possible.
- Look out for additives on food labels.
- Avoid refined and processed foods. Those that come in cans, jars and packets almost certainly contain additives (except for most foods purchased in health food stores). Fresh foods, on the other hand, are usually additive-free.
- Try to avoid caffeine, chocolate, cola drinks, alcohol and smoking. They may be enjoyable, but are especially detrimental in fibromyalgia.
- Avoid drinking at least half and hour before and half an hour after eating. Liquid dilutes the nutritional value of food.
- Due to the high fiber content of the fibromyalgia healing diet, try to drink 8 to 10 glasses of water a day, including fruit and vegetable juices and herbal teas. Distilled or filtered water is highly recommended.
- Be sure you are not consuming large quantities of salt. Remember that it is commonly used as a preservative and added to most processed, prepackaged foods. I recommend that you use minimal amounts in cooking and at the table. Rock salt, sea salt and natural seasonings are healthier alternatives, but should still be used sparingly.

- Take the recommended vitamin and mineral supplements. Because people with fibromyalgia suffer many nutritional deficiencies, tablet-form concentrates of a particular vitamin, mineral etc. are essential. Some nutritional supplements are required in high doses for a few months, after which a small maintenance dose should be taken.
- Take antioxidant supplements to protect the cells and to help the release of energy.

The following pages describe the recommended day-to-day diet for people with fibromyalgia, including the supplements known to be useful in treating the condition and outline a 21-day detoxification program that will help the body to eliminate stored toxins and debris. I advise, however, that you gradually accustom yourself to the new foods in this diet, that you get used to eating cleanly grown produce and additive-free foods for at least a month prior to embarking on the detoxification program. This will give your body and tastebuds time to adjust to the changes in your diet and minimize any possible side effects arising from detoxification.

8

Necessary Foods

The foods necessary for the treatment of fibromyalgia include:

- protein
- carbohydrate
- fat
- fiber

These essential nutrients provide our bodies with vital energy and, as our bodies are in a constant state of regeneration, serve as fundamental building materials.

It may not surprise you to know that junk or fast food is not recommended for people with fibromyalgia—or for healthy people for that matter. Individuals can survive on junk food for a while because it is comprised mainly of carbohydrates and fat, which have a high energy value. However, because junk food is short of sustaining nutrients, the body will not continue to repair and regenerate indefinitely. It slowly becomes clogged up, like a cog wheel that is fed pancake syrup instead of oil.

Our bodies also need a regular input of enzymes to function at optimum levels. Enzymes are crucial to good digestion, and many of them are provided by fresh raw food. Enzymes speed up the chemical reactions within our bodies and are essential to good health. Without sufficient enzymes, we deprive ourselves of the necessary nutrients. It is important to know that enzymes are easily destroyed in cooking and processing, so it is advisable to eat two to four portions of *raw* fruit and vegetables each day.

In total, we should try to consume five portions of fruit and five portions of vegetables a day, as recommended by the World Health Organization. Each of the following is equivalent to one portion:

- 4 ounces of a very large fruit; such as watermelon, melon or pineapple;
- a large fruit, such as an orange, banana or apple;
- 2 medium fruits, such as kiwi fruit and plums;
- 3 fluid ounces freshly squeezed fruit or vegetable juice;
- 4 ounces berries or cherries;
- a large bowl of salad;
- 3½ ounces (cooked weight) green vegetables;
- 3 ounces (cooked weight) root vegetables such as carrot or rutabaga, but do not include potatoes, sweet potatoes or yams;
- 3 ounces—cooked weight—small vegetables such as peas or sweet corn;
- 3 ounces of legumes or beans.

Of equal importance is that our diets contain sufficient roughage. This fibrous and bulking content of foods reduces the transit time of substances within the bowel. However, roughage is lost in food that has been refined. Thus, instead of being rapidly eliminated, refined food can sit in the bowel for much longer than it should, the resulting toxicity being reabsorbed into the body as it putrefies and rots there.

Protein

Our bodies are constructed of protein, so a good, steady supply is essential. Protein is vital to tissue regeneration and maintenance. It is also largely responsible for the production of hormones and the cells involved in immunity.

Digestive enzymes are required for protein synthesis, the transforming of proteins into repair constituents, which are used for cell regeneration. We need 22 amino acids, 14 of which can be produced by the body. The remaining 8 must be supplied by our food. All 22 amino acids are required at the same time and in the right quantity for protein synthesis. If just one is in short supply, the production of protein will be much reduced. It may even cease altogether. We have, therefore, a vital rationale for the consumption of sufficient protein-containing foods.

It may surprise you to know that a vegetarian diet that does not contain sufficient grain can cause protein foods to synthesize to form *carbohydrate* instead of protein—any excess carbohydrate being converted to fat. However, animal protein—meat, chicken, fish, dairy produce and eggs—contains all the essential amino acids and is the *only* source of vitamin B_{12}. Unfortunately, animal protein contains no fiber— an essential ingredient of the fibromyalgia healing diet. Instead, it can be loaded with saturated fat and cholesterol, which have a negative effect on the body. For these reasons, the fibromyalgia healing diet specifies only a small amount of animal protein. Dairy products should be consumed in moderation, too.

Fibromyalgia-friendly sources of protein are lean red meat, poultry, fish, tuna, soy products (all of which should be served in reasonably small helpings), cottage cheese, seeds, nuts and legumes. In a week, a serving of meat or fish no larger than the palm of your hand should be eaten on two to three occasions, two to three organic, free-range eggs should be consumed and butter should be spread very thinly on your whole-grain bread or rye crispbreads. In place of cows' milk, use soy milk, which is rich in protein, or rice milk, which has a high carbohydrate content. Goat's milk is an acceptable alternative, too.

Although vegetables and fruits are rich in fiber, carbohydrate and certain vitamins and minerals, they are low in protein. Nuts and legumes are excellent sources of protein, but must be combined to achieve a full range of amino acids, for example brown rice and lentils. However, a diet comprised mainly of nuts and legumes would render the individual vitamin B_{12} deficient.

It is a fact that people who eat a lot of grain products—bread, pasta, rice, cereals and so on—in an effort to limit their fat intake are likely to be consuming insufficient protein. This can lead to weakening of the immune system, which is suppressed in fibromyalgia anyway. If protein intake is low, the body will pull protein from the muscles, which then has the effect of slowing down the metabolism (the rate of conversion of food to energy). Protein deficiency causes low energy, low stamina, weakness, poor resistance to infection, depression and slow healing of wounds.

The consequences of a high-protein diet being uncertain, an interesting study into the effects of different quantities of protein intake was conducted in 2000.[11] It showed, surprisingly, that a high-protein diet can improve antioxidant status. However, it is now commonly known that a very high intake of protein may cause the tissues to be overly acidic, which can promote degenerative disease. Protein deficiency, on the other hand, causes oxidative stress, with the result that the immune system is weakened and inflammatory disorders of the arthritic type are likely to arise. I would advise, therefore, that approximately 20 to 25 percent of your total daily calories consist of protein.

Please do not worry too much about percentages, however. If you at least try to consume the recommended amounts of meat, as well as fruit, vegetables, nuts, seeds, legumes, soft-boiled egg yolks, soy products and so on, you will be doing your body a great favor. Remember, too, that healing changes will come about even if you are not able to follow this diet to the letter. Simply do the best you can and appreciate the fact that you are helping your body to fight this disease.

Although I do not advocate counting calories in the fibromyalgia healing diet, the following calorific values should give you a rough idea of not only your protein intake but also of your total calorific consumption (examples of carbohydrate and fat calories are given later in this chapter). Depending on your levels of activity—you are not likely to be very active if you are in a lot of pain—you should be eating between 1800 and 3000 calories a day.

Here are the calorific contents of some common protein foods:

- 1 ounce of grilled haddock—a very small piece—provides 40 calories;
- 1 ounce of roasted chicken—also a very small piece—provides 40 calories;
- 1 ounce of cottage cheese provides 15 calories;
- 1 ounce of Parmesan cheese provides 120 calories;
- 1 ounce of soy beans provides 50 calories.
- 1 ounce of butter provides 226 calories—so, to reiterate, butter should be used very sparingly.

Soy Products

The reduced activity levels common in people with fibromyalgia can lead to the early onset of osteoporosis. This is particularly likely among postmenopausal women. However, soy foods are believed to contain plant estrogen—estrogen being one of the hormones that are in short supply during and after menopause. These have the effect of preventing bone density loss and reducing hot flashes, irritability, aching joints and depression—all of which are symptoms of menopause. During a study in 2001, Japanese researchers concluded that the postmenopausal women who had consumed the highest amounts of soy-containing foods—such as tofu, soy milk and boiled soy beans—had increased bone mass and fewer backaches and aching joints than those who had consumed less of such foods.[12]

I would like to add a word of warning, however. Although rich in protein and very nutritious, high levels of soy consumption can suppress thyroid function. Because soy acts as a hormone in the body, it can interact with the delicate balance of thyroxine—the hormone produced by the thyroid gland. Consuming large amounts of soy products is capable of disrupting the thyroid gland, causing hypothyroidism (the state where thyroid levels are consistently too low). Pre-existing hypothyroidism may also be worsened.

My advice is, then, to drink no more than one glass of soy milk a day, maybe substituting a glass of rice milk later on. Other soy products, such as tofu, boiled soybeans and textured soy meats (sometimes called textured vegetable proteins—TVP) should be eaten on not more than one occasion every other day.

Carbohydrates

Carbohydrates—foods such as fruits, vegetables and grains (whole-grain bread, pasta, brown rice, cereals, couscous, millet, barley, bulgar wheat and so on)—supply our bodies with energy. Our digestive systems break down carbohydrates into simple sugars that are used to fuel essential body processes, such as brain function, nervous system function and muscle activity—all of which are problem areas in fibromyalgia. Any excess carbohydrate is converted to fat by insulin, the "fat-storage" hormone.

To guarantee the production of sufficient energy and ensure that fats and proteins are effectively broken down, we need to eat plenty of "complex" carbohydrates. These include fruits, vegetables, whole-grain breads, whole-grain pastas, brown rice, potatoes and sweet corn. "Simple" carbohydrates are the sugars found in table sugar, sweets, cakes and sweetened cereals. They provide a spurt of energy, but, in the long term, can cause blood sugar levels to fluctuate erratically. Simple carbohydrates should, therefore, be avoided as much as possible.

I reiterate that we should all try to eat five portions of fruit and five portions of vegetables a day, remembering that raw vegetables offer greater nutritional value than those that have been cooked. Organically grown fruit and vegetables are highly recommended—"organic" meaning grown without the presence of chemical pesticides and other toxins. Cleanly grown produce can now be found on our supermarket shelves and it is generally not much higher in price than chemically treated and grown foods.

As approximately half of our calorie intake should consist of carbohydrates, the calorific values of some recommended sources are as follows:

- 1 ounce of banana provides 22 calories;
- 1 ounce of orange provides 12 calories;
- 1 ounce of apple provides 17 calories;
- 1 ounce of whole-grain pasta provides 35 calories;
- 1 ounce of whole-grain bread provides 38 calories;
- 1 ounce of cauliflower provides 3 calories;
- 1 ounce of cabbage provides 4 calories.

Fats and Lipids (Oils)

Unfortunately, it is a fallacy that the answer to losing weight is simply to cut down on fat. Fats (fatty acids) are the most concentrated sources of energy in our diet—1 gram of fat providing the body with 9 calories of energy. Fat-containing foods are crucial to health as they slow the absorption of carbohydrates into the bloodstream, thus limiting the production of insulin, which is essential for controlling blood sugar levels. (Glucose, or blood sugar, is one of our body's most important nutrients and the basic source of energy for mind and body.)

There are two types of fats.

- **Saturated fats** These come mainly from animal sources and are generally solid at room temperature. For many years, margarine was believed to be a healthier choice than butter. However, it is now known that some of the fats in the hydrogenation process involved in making margarine are changed into trans-fatty acids, and the body metabolizes them as if they were saturated fatty acids—the same as butter. Although butter should be used sparingly, it is also a valuable source of oils and vitamin A. Margarine, on the other hand, is an artificial product containing many additives and should be avoided.

- **Unsaturated fats** These are often called "polyunsaturated" or "monounsaturated" fats and are derived mainly from vegetables, nuts and seeds. They are usually liquid at room temperature. Examples of unsaturated fats are olive, canola, safflower and sunflower oils.

While saturated fats are believed to be implicated in the development of heart disease, unsaturated fats actually have a *protective* effect. Omega 3 and omega 6 fatty acids are obtained from vegetable oils, seeds (sunflower seeds, sesame seeds, flaxseeds and so on), nuts, avocados and oily fish (salmon, mackerel, herring, tuna and others).

Olive oil is considered the superior source of these acids because it suffers less damage during cooking than other oils. All oils should be stored in sealed containers in a cool, dark place to prevent the onset of rancidity.

Oils are a natural source of vitamin E, which is an important antioxidant. Antioxidants are essential to cell life because they mop up destructive "free radicals" within the body. Unfortunately, during processing, the vitamin E in some unsaturated oils is removed, depriving the body of this vitamin. Processed oils are also very susceptible to rancidity. It is recommended, therefore, that you obtain your fats from natural sources, including cold-pressed vegetable oils.

It is important to note that the process of frying changes the molecular structure of foods, rendering them potentially damaging to the body. If you must fry something, it is best to use a small amount of extra virgin olive oil and cook at a low temperature. Sautéing in a little water or tomato juice can be quite acceptable, but, otherwise, grilling, baking and steaming are better alternatives. A word of warning—never reheat used oils, for this, too, can be harmful to the body.

You have probably heard that eggs are high in cholesterol, which is a type of fat. There is, however, little conclusive evidence to support the theory that dietary cholesterol can lead to heart disease. Eggs are also known to contain lecithin, which is a superb biological "detergent" that is capable of breaking down fats so they can be used by the body. Eggs should be soft-boiled or poached, as a hard yolk will bind the lecithin, rendering it useless as a "fat detergent." Although I have recommended that you eat two to three eggs a week, those following the fibromyalgia healing diet on a vegetarian basis should eat up to five eggs a week to obtain the necessary protein.

It is estimated that the fat intake of most adults is 42 percent of their total daily calories, and that this figure mostly consists of saturated fat. However, the recommended daily intake is 20 percent—1 ounce, which amounts to only 270 calories. Eating the necessary unsaturated fats will ensure reduced calorie intake and greater energy provision.

Here are the caloric values of some fat-containing foods:

- 1 ounce of oil contains 130 calories;
- 1 ounce of butter contains 226 calories;
- 1 ounce of eggs contains 80 calories;
- 1 ounce of oily fish contains 60 calories.

Fiber (Roughage)

A type of carbohydrate, fiber is the indigestible parts of plants. It is the cellulose fibers forming the leaf webbing in green vegetables, it is the skins of sweet corn and beans, and it is the husks of wheat and corn. Foods containing fiber include fruits, vegetables, nuts, seeds, beans, peas, lentils, whole-grain breads and cereals (wheat, oats, rye, barley, corn and so on). In fact, a large percentage of the foods recommended in the fibromyalgia healing diet contain fiber, and the above-mentioned are all highly nutritious foods, providing not only fiber but also starch and many essential vitamins and minerals.

One of the most compelling reasons that fiber has become popular in weight-loss programs is because the appetite is satiated on far fewer calories. This important food constituent also ensures slower and more regulated absorption of glucose into the bloodstream. As a result, you avoid plummeting into hunger troughs and craving sugars to raise blood sugar levels.

Nutritionists have labeled fiber "nature's broom" because it quickly sweeps the system clean, ensuring no unhealthy waste products lurk in hidden corners. When waste persistently lingers in the bowel, as happens in low-fiber diets, immune system disorders often result. Fibromyalgia is one such disorder.

A moderately high fiber intake will, therefore, speed up the transit time of material in the large intestine, limiting the amount of toxins absorbed back into the bloodstream from the digestive tract. As toxicity and irritable bowel syndrome are both linked to fibromyalgia, I recommend that each meal have some fiber content. Furthermore, because of the bulking capacity of fiber, high levels of water consumption are necessary. I recommend, that eight to 10 glasses of water—including the liquid in fruit and vegetable drinks and herbal teas—should be drunk daily. The water in coffee and tea (even decaffeinated), caffeinated soft drinks and alcohol does not count. Drinks containing caffeine are diuretics and actually make the body lose fluid. Alcohol can lead to dehydration, too.

Salt

Although our bodies need the sodium we obtain from salt, high intakes of it have a detrimental effect in many ways. High blood pressure and heart disease are only two conditions that are commonly linked to diets high in salt. A food additive, salt is used in virtually all processed foods as a preservative as it has the capacity to inhibit the growth of harmful micro-organisms. It is also added in large amounts to most breakfast cereals, except for shredded wheat products and a few others.

I would recommend that small amounts of sea or rock salt be used in baking, that a small amount of this mineral-rich salt be added to cooking, but that you try to avoid sprinkling any type of salt over your meals. Gradually reducing your intake of salt is the best way to retrain your palate.

The only exception to this rule is that people in hot climates and those who sweat a lot should make sure that lost salt is always replaced, since sweating causes sodium levels to drop.

9

Why Diet Is Important in Treating Fibromyalgia

I'd had trouble with my stomach for so long! Allergy testing suggested that yeast intolerance was my problem. Then some of my fellow fibromyalgics had tests. What a surprise! Most of them had yeast-related problems, too!

In addition, people with fibromyalgia suffer from the following:

- suppressed immune systems;
- the processing of nerve sensations is confused;
- certain hormone levels are abnormal;
- the soft tissues (muscles, tendons and ligaments) are low in energy and clogged with waste materials.

Proper diet can help remedy all of these conditions, but only if the digestive process is functioning effectively. There is, undoubtedly, a lot to be corrected!

Diet and the Digestive System

A breakdown in the functions and processes within the digestive system is frequently found in fibromyalgia. In fact, many experts are now of the opinion that impaired digestion is actually one of the chief causes of the condition.

The factors leading to a digestive system breakdown may include stress and anxiety, eating too quickly, inadequate chewing, toxicity problems, the effects of antibiotic medications and a poor diet.

Abnormal intestinal microflora

Full health of the digestive system depends on an individual having ecologically "balanced" gut microflora—the bacteria that help to break down foods. Friendly bacteria not only aid digestion, they also protect against invaders such as the parasitic yeast infection known as candida. The fact that many people with fibromyalgia suffer from chronic yeast infections is becoming more and more apparent. (See Chapter 2.)

Candidiasis is an infection that is caused by the candida fungus, usually of the candida albicans variety. In otherwise healthy people, candida infections are rarely serious, but when the immune system is depressed for some reason, candida can become a real problem. Some evidence suggests that it can also be induced by coming off sleeping pills and tranquilizers after prolonged usage. Many experts also firmly believe that candidiasis can occur after a gastric infection, particularly when the patient has taken a course of antibiotics to treat the upset.

Candida overgrowth (candidiasis)

Everyone has resident microflora in the gut that are capable of fermenting dietary sugars. It is only when the balance is upset and this type of microflora remains that fermentation actually takes place. When fermenting organisms are allowed to occupy a large area of the gut they multiply rapidly, producing alcohol and other toxins. Large overgrowths of candida can cause unsteadiness, clumsiness and slurred speech. The presence of this type of yeast infection can also interfere with the absorption of important nutrients into the bloodstream.

Candida does not arise as a result of *all* microorganism fermentation, but it is a very common cause. However, when the candida is eliminated and balanced gut microflora restored, the individual is often relieved of many of the symptoms tied in with both fibromyalgia and irritable bowel syndrome (IBS).

THE SYMPTOMS OF CANDIDA OVERGROWTH

Excessive amounts of intestinal candida can cause abdominal bloating and discomfort, alternating bouts of constipation and diarrhea (or just diarrhea), flatulence, indigestion, fatigue, depression, poor concentration, headaches (including migraine attacks), short-term memory problems, joint and muscle pains, and disturbed sleep—most of which are the primary symptoms of fibromyalgia!

When candida is eradicated and steps taken to ensure it does not recur, the symptoms of fibromyalgia can greatly recede. (There is no evidence, as yet, to suggest that they *totally* disappear.)

INTESTINAL FERMENTATION

It is now known that when there is an overgrowth of candida, fermentation products are absorbed into the bloodstream. Tests have shown that blood alcohol levels rise significantly within an hour of the affected person eating sugar. When absorbed into the blood, these toxins (fermentation products) travel to the brain where ensuing adverse function can give rise to fatigue, depression, disturbed sleep, headaches and memory problems. As observed above, in some people, the candida overgrowth is so great they really can be mistaken for being drunk!

YEAST TOXINS

With the progression of the yeast infection (that is, the overgrowth of candida), toxins are released into the bowel, from whence they again are absorbed into the bloodstream and this produces further symptoms. Some of these toxins have the effect of suppressing the immune system, some induce allergic reactions and others generate the production of antibodies that react against healthy tissues. In this instance, the ovaries may be attacked, causing premenstrual syndrome, irregular periods, reduced libido and so on, or the thyroid gland may be rendered inactive, with significant consequences.

A suppressed immune system, allergies and tissue damage are conditions often found in fibromyalgia. In fact, some experts in the field believe a suppressed immune system to be one of the major causes of the condition.

YEAST ALLERGY

In addition, we now also know that the immune system can set up antibodies to the yeast organism itself. When this occurs, allergic reactions within the bowel can arise and allergic conditions, such as asthma and urticara (an allergic skin rash) may develop. People affected will react against all foods containing yeast, as well as foods that advance yeast fermentation, such as sugar, alcohol and caffeine.

Permeability of the intestinal wall

In a healthy person, food is thoroughly digested before its products are absorbed into the bloodstream. Food will not slip through the bowel wall until the digestive enzymes have broken it down into minuscule units. Our immune systems do not recognize these units as foreign, simply because our bodies are made of the same basic building blocks as the foods we eat. However, when the gut wall is significantly damaged by fermentation products and allergic reactions to yeast overgrowth, food molecules are able to escape into the bloodstream before they have been properly digested.

Because these molecules are larger than usual—they are called macromolecules—the immune system recognizes them as foreign and so sets up antibodies to fight them. All healthy people absorb some of these macromolecules, but, because they are in relatively small amounts, the immune system can normally cope.

One theory about what happens next is that when vast amounts of these macromolecules are absorbed, the immune system, confused by the constant onslaught, begins to attack the body's own cells—the muscles, ligaments and so on—by mistake. It then sets up antibodies to foods other than yeasts and the body thus develops food intolerances.

By now you are probably wondering, how can you know for sure whether or not you have a yeast problem? In addition to the many symptoms outlined previously, a craving for sugar can be a good indication. Fermenting microbes thrive on sugar, therefore the individual affected can feel somewhat sugar deficient and, as a result, eat more sweet foods, which feed the yeast. Thus a vicious circle prevails. (Sugar cravings can also point to hypoglycemia, a condition requiring urgent attention from your doctor. It is important, therefore, never to make assumptions about your health. Informing your doctor of all your health worries is essential.) Yeast problems are also indicated by recurrent bouts of oral, or, in women, vaginal, thrush.

You may wish to undergo allergy testing, as an in-patient at a special clinic or by asking your doctor to send off blood samples to a testing lab or by visiting designated premises for evaluation by a "sensor" machine (although there is some doubt about the accuracy of the latter).

Note that, although you may present yourself for allergy testing, the tester will actually look for the foods to which you are sensitive.

THE YEASTS IN OUR ENVIRONMENT

Yeasts are a group of microscopic fungi that exist in many different environments in nature. They may be present in our diet deliberately, as in baking and fermentation, or accidentally, as in overripe fruit and food that has been left lying around for too long. As sugar encourages the growth of yeast, removing all forms of sugar is recommended for individuals with a chronic yeast infection. Also, as sufferers are often sensitive to yeast itself, all yeast products should be removed, too.

The Elimination Program

Discovering whether or not you are sensitive to a particular type of food can be very difficult, and each of the tests available can be criticized if you deliberately set out to do so. The only certain way to prove the case is via a food elimination program, but to eliminate one food at a time, then to have to wait in order to assess your body's response, would take many months to do. For this reason, attending an allergy-testing clinic is advisable. The results will at least point you in the right direction. Also, there are many allergy-friendly foods and supplements available in health food stores and pharmacies.

Does food elimination have side effects?

Assuming that the foods eliminated were the right ones to start with, there is often an initial withdrawal reaction. Fatigue, headaches, twitching and irritability are normal symptoms, and can persist for up to 15 days. Drinking at least 5 pints of water helps to reduce such symptoms. It also aids detoxification, helping to flush any residual offending foods through the system.

A hypersensitive stage can then follow this period. If the person has unwittingly eaten a food they are attempting to eliminate, the ensuing reaction can be severe, particularly when there is a true allergy. Dining out can be a problem, too. Ask the chef, not the waiter, if you are unsure about ingredients.

On a brighter note, a pleasing withdrawal symptom can be weight loss. The reason for this effect—assuming you are not starving yourself, which would be completely wrong and unnecessary—is that many people with food sensitivities have an unrecognized excess of fluid distributed throughout their bodies. When they begin to eliminate certain suspect foods, then start to feel better, the excess fluid quickly drains away.

It is important to note that a yeast-free diet will normally reduce the intake of calcium, protein, fiber, fat and B vitamins—all of which are obtained in a normal diet. However, this problem can be rectified by increasing consumption of cereals, vegetables, liver, fish—and by taking the allergy-friendly B group of vitamins. All fruit should be thoroughly washed first, dried, then peeled and eaten immediately.

Elimination and reintroduction strategy

Should you wish to discover whether or not you have a yeast problem without going to the trouble and expense of allergy testing, try avoiding and keeping to the foods in Table 1 for a period of one month.

In addition, drinks and foods that contain caffeine (coffee, tea, chocolate, cola) should be avoided. These products induce a quick sugar-

TABLE 1: Foods to avoid in identifying yeast intolerance		
FOODS TO AVOID		ALTERNATIVES
Cheese (including cottage and cream)	Spirits	Perhaps the most difficult yeast food to replace is bread. However, health food stores now stock a sugar, yeast, wheat, egg and milk-free bread mix, to which you just add the flour of your choice. There are also soda bread, soda bread mixes, chapatis, matzos, water biscuits, rye crispbreads and rice cakes.
Ordinary bread	Monosodium glutamate (MSG)	
Cakes	Mushrooms	
Pita bread and buns	Soy sauce	
Boullion cubes	Tartar sauce	
Vinegar		
Pickles	Watch out for "leavening," "pickled" "fermented" and "malt" on labels.	
Beer		
Wine		
Cider		
Dried fruits	Chocolate containing sugar	For broth, use homemade, kept frozen, or vegetable bouillon paste or cubes, broth mix or soy cubes—all made without yeast.
Yogurt		
Salad dressings		
Ketchup	Removing all forms of sugar is recommended.	
Stuffing		
Tofu		

TABLE 2: Things to avoid if you are sensitive to fungi	
PLACES THAT HARBOR WATER	
Cheese (including cottage and cream)	Woodpiles
Damp towels and clothing	Roofs leaking into attics or behind walls
Old peeling wallpaper and paste	
Pet litter	Shower curtains
Vaporizers	Rubbish bins
Potted plants	Vegetable bins
Leather goods	Old mattresses
Paint that is peeling	Leaky pipes and taps
Overstuffed furniture	Refrigerator drip trays and rubber door gaskets
Foam rubber pillows	
Hay and grain fields	Compost piles or leaf piles
Poorly ventilated closets	Damp or flooded basements

release that is not desirable where yeast has proliferated. If possible, try to avoid alcohol, too. It may be difficult when you are with other people. The thing to remember is not to be obsessive about it, just careful.

Make sure you are eating enough "staple foods." Cutting down too much can lead to nutritional deficiencies.

Individuals who have an intolerance to yeast will also be sensitive to fungi—that is, molds and mildew. The list in Table 2 gives examples of possible causes of asthma and chronic rhinitis.

Reintroducing excluded foods

Toward the end of the month, many of you should feel better than you have for a long time! The feeling of well-being can be so great you won't want to bother to reintroduce the foods you excluded.

However, for those who do wish to reintroduce those foods, the following procedure is suggested.

Day 1	In the morning, reintroduce a small amount of a food or drink previously eliminated (not a full-sized portion). Do the same later in the day. Record any symptoms.

Day 2	If you fail to experience symptoms, repeat the exercise. Once again, record any symptoms. If you get through the second day, this is really good news! Well done!
Days 3 and 4	Wait for two days before you can safely reintroduce this food into your diet on a fairly regular basis.
Thereafter	Repeat the above four-day reintroduction procedure with each food eliminated.

Any side effects should have occurred within four days. You may be disappointed, however, if your problem is not intolerance but true allergy. True allergies cause an immediate reaction—the immune system responds as if it is being invaded, thereby setting up antibodies to the offending food(s). Obviously you will need to continue to avoid this food.

If you do experience symptoms—for example, you develop a headache after reintroducing cheese—it would be better to leave cheese alone for at least six months before attempting to reintroduce it again. Some foods will always cause an adverse reaction, so it would be wise to withdraw them from your diet altogether.

In the meantime, continue to eat sensibly. Try not to indulge too much in the foods that previously caused problems. Remember—if in doubt, leave it out!

Lack of vitamin and mineral absorption

Slow absorption may be the underlying problem in people who have multiple food sensitivities or true allergies. This usually means that essential vitamins and minerals are slow to be absorbed too and, consequently, the person will suffer deficiencies. This particularly applies to the water-soluble B group and C vitamins.

The individual will probably also have deficiencies in important minerals, such as magnesium, calcium, potassium, zinc and iron. In short, a person with multiple food sensitivities/allergies and so on should probably take multivitamin and multimineral supplements on a long-term basis. Your doctor's advice should be sought first, however.

Amino Acids

The components that affect all of the above-mentioned systems and processes are amino acids, which are known as "the building blocks of life." Their functions include cell manufacture, muscle and tissue repair and the manufacture of antibodies. A total of 22 amino acids are capable of being produced when protein is broken down by the digestive process, 8 of these being essential because they cannot be manufactured by the body. With proper nutrition, the remaining 14 can be manufactured, however.

Although no studies have yet been conducted some experts are of the opinion that a certain branch chain of amino acids holds the key to the cause and treatment of fibromyalgia. The chain in question includes amino acids called "tryptophan" and "tyrosine," both of which are transported through the gut by the same protein molecule. People with fibromyalgia are known to have reduced levels of these two amino acids. In fact, tryptophan and tyrosine are now known to be especially susceptible to damage by toxicity and it is becoming increasingly evident that fibromyalgia can arise as a result of toxicity problems.

Below is a description of the affected amino acids, together with a corrective treatment.

- **Tryptophan** Tryptophan produces serotonin, which is known to be deficient in fibromyalgia. Tryptophan-rich foods include fish, turkey, chicken, avocados, bananas, cottage cheese and wheat germ. However, when the tryptophan carrier molecule is damaged, as is believed to be the case in fibromyalgia, the aforementioned foods may not be converted into serotonin. 5-Hydroxy-tryptophan (5-HTP), though, is capable of successfully raising serotonin levels. This enzyme, which is available as a supplement from health food stores, does not have the side effects that often arise with pharmaceutical serotonin-enhancing medications, so it can be a valuable alternative to them. The recommended daily dose for fibromyalgics is 100 to 500 mg, depending on the severity of symptoms. It should be taken an hour before bedtime with a carbohydrate food, such as whole-grain toast, rice or oat cakes, rye crispbread and so on, to encourage improved sleep. I would, however, strongly advise that you consult your doctor before taking this supplement.

- **Tyrosine**   This important amino acid is the precursor to the thyroid hormones. It is involved in the transmission of nerve impulses to the brain; improving memory; increasing mental alertness and promoting healthy functioning of the thyroid gland. Long-term improvements in the symptoms of fibromyalgia have been seen as a result of electro-acupuncture, which works in exactly the same way as conventional acupuncture, except that electrical stimulation is used in place of needles. A TENS (Transcutaneous Electronic Nerve Stimulation) machine with surface electrodes, used for 30 minutes twice to seven times a week, can also be effective. Your local physical therapy department may be able to provide further information.

We have known for several years that stress and/or physical trauma from, for example, a traffic accident or surgery, can trigger fibromyalgia. These events may also damage certain amino acids. In fact, emotional and physical trauma are thought to play a leading role in not only altering amino acids but also in increasing the levels of the stress hormones.

Other Possible Causes

Overly high stress hormone levels are capable of irritating and inflaming the intestinal lining, causing it to not function properly. The intestinal lining is intended only to allow the absorption of nutrients into the bloodstream, while keeping back toxins. Where stress hormones have indirectly caused damage to the intestinal lining, toxins are able to leak into the bloodstream. Cortisol, for example, one of the main stress hormones, interferes with sleep, which in turn has the effect of reducing the body's ability to repair the intestine. The immune system then sends out antibodies to gobble up toxins it does not recognize, which may simply be large particles of food. In fibromyalgia, the immune system appears to be permanently on overdrive to deal with the leaked toxins—a weakened immune system being the eventual result.

Where fibromyalgia develops gradually over many years, as occurs in some cases, genetic factors are believed to be responsible, in addition to borderline function of the amino acid transport proteins. When amino acid transport is further damaged by junk food diets, environmental chemicals, chronic exposure to the low-level toxicity found in food additives, as well as mercury vapor from amalgam tooth fillings, fibromyalgia can arise.

However, fibromyalgia symptoms are known to recede when the intestines are cleaned up. The cleansing process chiefly consists of:

- a detoxification program;
- an additive-free diet;
- antioxidant-containing foods and supplementation.

10

Essential Nutrients

There are many nutrients essential to good health, ones that support the repair and regeneration of the tissues and cells. They fall into several categories, including vitamins, minerals, essential fatty acids, amino acids and enzymes. Enzymes are made up of vitamins and minerals and act as powerful antioxidants.

Antioxidants

Unfortunately, oxygen is not always a beneficial agent. A car needs a mixture of oxygen and fuel to run, but it is oxygen that plays a crucial role in the rusting process, shortening the life of the vehicle. Oxygen is essential to many functions within living organisms, too, and, like rust to the car, the presence of electrically unstable oxygen atoms within our bodies can seriously affect our health and longevity.

These unstable oxygen atoms—known as "free radicals"—run riot around our bodies, damaging cell walls and important DNA. Researchers have found that disease is directly influenced by the number of free radicals present in an individual. In some instances, free radicals will cause disease, in others they will exacerbate a pre-existing illness. Antioxidants are important because they mop up free radicals.

As people with fibromyalgia are burdened with a large supply of destructive free radicals—a situation known as "oxidative stress"—it is vital that plenty of antioxidant-containing foods, supplemented with antioxidant nutrients, are consumed. Many vitamins and minerals contain antioxidant properties, each type having its own working domain and mode of operation. The best vitamin sources include selenium, vitamin A, vitamin C and vitamin E. Good antioxidant foods are garlic, turmeric and canola extract products (proanthocyanidins).

Smoking cigarettes or cigars greatly increases free radical damage. Smokers having low levels of antioxidant nutrients in their bodies. Although antioxidants, taken daily, can reduce free radical damage, the best option is to give up smoking.

Another positive benefit of consuming the recommended daily amount of antioxidants is a longer life. When bombarded with free radicals, our cells become depleted of energy, a situation that commonly leads to chronic disease such as fibromyalgia. Eventually, the attacked cells die, which is detrimental to the individual. However, antioxidants enable our cells to be more productive, effectively preventing cell death.

In order to secure optimum functioning of each of the millions of cells in our bodies, it is important to protect them by means of a steady intake of antioxidant foods and nutritional supplements.

Vitamins

Unlike proteins, carbohydrates and fats, vitamins do not provide energy or act as building materials. Their chief function is to sustain and regulate certain biochemical processes, including cellular reproduction, digestion and the metabolic rate.

Vitamins are organic food substances found only in plants and animals. They are essential to the normal functioning of our bodies, so we must make sure that our intake of them is adequate. However, due to the use of chemicals in the production of crops, it is difficult to acquire sufficient amounts, even from a good-quality, balanced diet. The common habit of overcooking vegetables leads to a further loss in their nutritional value. In addition, people with fibromyalgia are known to suffer multiple vitamin deficiencies. It is important, therefore, that vitamin supplements be taken daily. These generally come in tablet or capsule form and can be purchased at health food stores. They should be taken before meals to ensure maximum absorption.

I have included the recommended daily allowance (RDAs) of both vitamins and minerals for people with fibromyalgia. Although they are rather higher than the government RDAs, the latter are meant only to prevent deficiency symptoms in healthy people. However, if you suffer adverse effects from taking the amounts recommended here for fibromyalgia, reduce the dose accordingly.

Vitamin C

One of the more potent antioxidants, vitamin C aids in maintaining healthy bones, teeth and gums; wound-healing; the absorption of iron in the intestines stress hormone production and immune system function.

Vitamin C is used up in the body by smoking, alcohol consumption, surgery, trauma, stress, exposure to pollutants and the use of certain medications.

Fibromyalgia-friendly food sources high in vitamin C are citrus fruits, strawberries, black currant, tomatoes, broccoli, Brussels sprouts, cabbage, green melons, potatoes and peppers (capsicums).

As this vitamin is easily destroyed by heat and processing, it is recommended that vegetables be steamed or microwaved for as short a period of time as possible.

Vitamin C deficiency is characterized by bleeding gums, swollen and/or painful joints, nosebleeds, loss of appetite, muscular weakness, slow-healing wounds, anemia and impaired digestion.

The government recommended daily amount (RDA) is 60 mg. However, the RDA for people with fibromyalgia is 1000 to 2000 mg.

Vitamin A (beta-carotene—the precursor to retinol)

Also a powerful antioxidant, vitamin A is necessary for the growth and repair of the body's tissues. In addition, it reduces susceptibility to infections in the nose, mouth, throat and lungs, aids bone and teeth formation, and helps to protect against pollutants.

Fibromyalgia-friendly food sources high in vitamin A are yellow and orange fruits and vegetables, such as carrots, sweet potatoes, apricots, cantaloupe, papaya, pumpkin, melon and mango. Beta-carotene can also be found in dark, leafy vegetables such as spinach, broccoli, cabbage and parsley.

Symptoms of deficiency are a susceptibility to infections; rough, dry, scaly skin; loss of smell and appetite; fatigue; defective teeth and gums; and retarded growth.

Vitamin A should not be taken during pregnancy.

The RDA is 3333 IUs for males and 2667 IUs for females. However, the RDA for fibromyalgia is 10,000 IUs.

Vitamin E

Another major antioxidant, vitamin E helps to supply oxygen to all the organs in the body, helping to alleviate fatigue. It also nourishes the cells, strengthens capillary walls, protects red blood cells from toxins and aids in the maintenance of nerve and muscle function.

As with other supplements, people taking warfarin should check with their doctor before taking vitamin E supplements.

Fibromyalgia-friendly food sources high in vitamin E are mostly oil, seed and grain derivatives. These include wheat germ, safflower, avocados, sunflower oil and seeds, pumpkin seeds, flaxseeds, almonds, Brazil nuts, cashews, pecans, whole-grain cereals and breads, wheat germ, asparagus, dried prunes and broccoli.

Symptoms of vitamin E deficiency are dry skin; red blood cell rupture; decline in sexual vitality; abnormal fat deposits in the muscles; degenerative changes in the heart and the muscles and the onset of autoimmune disease (fibromyalgia is an autoimmune disease—"autoimmune" means that the immune system is confused into attacking healthy tissues, such as the muscles, ligaments and tendons).

The RDA is 10 mg, but, for those with fibromyalgia, it is 250 mg.

B complex vitamins

As the B vitamins are required at every stage of energy manufacture, and because they assist in the calming process and in maintaining good mental health, a regular intake is required in the treatment of fibromyalgia. B vitamins are also integral to the production of serotonin, the pain-reducing, sleep-promoting hormone that fibromyalgics have in short supply. For all these reasons, B complex vitamin supplements are highly recommended for people with fibromyalgia. Avoid taking them at night, however, as they may interfere with sleep.

VITAMIN B$_1$ (THIAMINE)

This vitamin is essential for blood cell metabolism; muscle metabolism; digestion; pain inhibition and energy production, all of which can be problem areas in fibromyalgia. In fact, fibromyalgics are known to exhibit a low vitamin B$_1$ status, causing reduced activity of the thiamine-dependent enzymes. A diet that is low in sugars and high in whole grains will improve vitamin B levels, however.

Fibromyalgia-friendly food sources high in vitamin B$_1$ are oatmeal, whole wheat, brown rice, bran, wheat germ, lentils, lean meats, free-range eggs, dried beans, sunflower seeds and peanuts. Herbs containing B$_1$ are peppermint, slippery elm, ginseng, gotu kola and kelp.

Deficiency problems include burning and tingling in the toes and soles of the feet, depression, fatigue, muscle weakness, difficulty sleeping, irritability and loss of appetite.

The RDA is 1.5 mg for males and 1.1 mg for females. However, the RDA for fibromyalgia is 30 mg.

VITAMIN B$_2$ (RIBOFLAVIN)

Necessary for red blood formation; cell respiration; antibody formation and fat and carbohydrate metabolism, the body should be supplied with vitamin B$_2$ daily. Levels of this vitamin in the body can be reduced by caffeine, alcohol and some antibiotics.

Fibromyalgia-friendly food sources high in vitamin B$_2$ are peanuts, free-range eggs, lean meats, soy products, whole grains and leafy green vegetables.

Deficiency symptoms include insomnia; dry, cracked lips; a red, scaly nose; gritty eyes, sore lips and tongue and photophobia (light-sensitive eyes).

The RDA is 1.7 mg for males and 1.3 mg for females. However, the RDA for fibromyalgia is 25 mg.

VITAMIN B$_3$ (NIACINAMIDE)

This vitamin is necessary for the production of several hormones, including insulin, female and male hormones and thyroxine, the hormone produced by the thyroid gland. It is also involved in blood circulation, acid production, histamine activation and conversion of carbohydrates to energy.

Fibromyalgia-friendly food sources high in vitamin B_3 are white meat, whole wheat, oily fish, avocados, nuts, peanuts, sunflower seeds, whole grains and prunes.

B_3 deficiency can cause hypoglycemia, confusion, memory loss, irritability, diarrhea, depression, fatigue, muscle weakness, insomnia and ringing in the ears.

The RDA is 1.1 mg. However, the RDA for fibromyalgia is 100 mg.

VITAMIN B_5 (PANTOTHENIC ACID)

The adrenal glands, which sit on top of the kidneys, can be damaged by stress, causing "adrenal exhaustion" and all manner of problems. Further damage can be prevented, however, by taking this supplement. B_5 is also crucial to the release of energy from protein, carbohydrates, fats and sugars; for the production of the anti-stress hormones and for good health of the nervous system.

Symptoms of deficiency include muscle pain; dizzy spells; skin abnormalities; digestive problems; poor muscle coordination, restlessness; fatigue, depression and insomnia.

Fibromyalgia-friendly food sources high in vitamin B_5 are whole grains, soft-boiled egg yolk, fish, brewer's yeast, peanuts, walnuts, dried pears and apricots, dates and mushrooms.

The RDA is 6 mg. However, the RDA for fibromyalgia is 50 mg.

VITAMIN B_6 (PYRIDOXINE)

Needed for the conversion of fats and proteins into energy, vitamin B_6 is vital for correct balance in the body and important for those who suffer excessive stress. It also aids in the production of serotonin, and is essential for magnesium metabolism—both of which fibromyalgics have in short supply.

Symptoms of B_6 deficiency include nervousness, depression, muscle weakness, pain, headaches, irritability, stiff joints and PMS in women.

Fibromyalgia-friendly food sources high in vitamin B_6 are bananas, whole-grain bread, lean meats, eggs, dried beans, avocados, seeds, nuts, chicken, fish and liver.

The RDA is 2 mg. Although the safety of vitamin B_6 supplementation has been under the spotlight in recent years, the fibromyalgia RDA of 50 mg is considered safe, even for long-term use.

VITAMIN B_{12} (COBALAMIN)

This vitamin is crucial to protein, carbohydrate and fat metabolism, red blood cell formation and longevity of cells. As B_{12} is found in animal products, supplementation is essential for vegans. Muscle weakness, fatigue, depression, paranoia, memory loss and headaches are symptoms of vitamin B_{12} deficiency.

Fibromyalgia-friendly food sources high in vitamin B_{12} are soft-boiled egg yolk, fish, shellfish, lean meats and poultry.

The RDA is 1 mcg. However, the RDA for fibromyalgia is 250 mcg.

Vitamin P (bioflavonoids and proanthocyanidins)

Because they work with vitamin C, bioflavonoids are essential for people with fibromyalgia. The condition means that the cells allow substances to leak through thin blood vessel walls to accumulate in tissues where they are not supposed to be. Natural plant bioflavonoids such as rutin, hesperidin and quercetin, help to strengthen the vessels and capillaries. High-potency bioflavonoids called "proanthocyanidins"—the most potent of which is canola extract (available from health food stores)—also strengthen the blood vessels and capillaries. Their other benefits include strengthening connective tissues and muscle fiber; enhancing muscle fiber function; improving the energy production process and reducing free radical damage. They also assist in utilizing other nutrients.

Although they are found in virtually all plant foods, the best fibromyalgia-friendly food sources high in bioflavonoids are fresh fruit and vegetables, legumes, whole grains, seeds, nuts, spinach, apricots, cherries, rosehips, grapes, blackberries and tea. Bioflavonoid-containing herbs include paprika and rosehips. Milk thistle seed, ginkgo biloba and pycnogenol (which is obtained from canola extract) are high in bioflavonoids and can be purchased in tablet form from health food stores and specialist suppliers.

There is no government RDA for bioflavonoids and proanthocyanidins as they are groups of nutrients. People with fibromyalgia should try to consume the above foods and take milk thistle and ginkgo biloba supplements, closely following the dosage instructions on the container.

Biotin

This vitamin reduces stress, aids nutrient absorption and is especially beneficial to individuals who eat a poor-quality diet. It helps protein, carbohydrate and fat metabolism; cell growth, fatty acid production and energy metabolism.

Biotin deficiency is characterized by muscle pain, fatigue, depression, nausea, anemia, hair loss, anorexia, dermatitis and high cholesterol levels.

Fibromyalgia-friendly food sources high in biotin are lean meats, soft-boiled egg yolk and whole grains.

The RDA is 150 mcg. However, the RDA for fibromyalgia is 400 mcg.

Minerals

Minerals are our most essential nutrients. The body requires small amounts of a wide range of minerals on a daily basis to ensure the normal functioning of all its systems. Carbohydrates, fats, vitamins, enzymes and amino acids all require minerals for their particular operations. However, one of their more important functions is that of aiding the regulation of the delicate balance of bodily fluids. They are also essential to the process of waste elimination and for bringing oxygen and nutrients to the cells.

As minerals continue to disappear from our soils, humans face an ongoing rise in mineral deficiencies. In addition, government studies have shown that prolonged stress and anxiety can lead to mineral imbalances, which is now considered a major factor in the onset of fibromyalgia.

People with fibromyalgia are known to have abnormally low levels of magnesium and manganese. Many sufferers also have other mineral deficiencies and, unfortunately, a shortage of essential minerals causes deficiencies in protein and vitamins. Besides eating a quality, well-balanced diet, it is imperative that people with fibromyalgia take mineral supplements. These usually come in tablet form and can be purchased at health food stores, pharmacies and most supermarkets.

It is important to be aware that all minerals are bound to something else, which is known as "chelation," and the amount of mineral absorbed by the body depends on what the mineral is chelated to.

"Inorganic chelates" are naturally occurring mined minerals that are not easily absorbed by the body. For example, women with osteoporosis may take calcium carbonate. However, its absorption may be as little as 5 percent—that's 50 mg from a 1000 mg supplement. Oxides, sulphates and phosphates are also inorganic chelates and may not be very useful.

"Organic chelates," on the other hand, can achieve up to 60 percent absorption. So, while the milligrams figure may be lower, the body will absorb far greater amounts. Check the label for the words "amino acid chelate," "citrate," "picolinate" or "glycinate," which indicate that the product is an organic chelate. Because organic chelated minerals are more expensive to produce, the cost to the consumer is greater than that of their inorganic counterparts. However, the cost is more than made up for by their far superior effects.

The following are important minerals:

Calcium

This vital mineral is the most abundant in the body—99 percent of it being found in the bones and teeth. Calcium works to tighten and constrict bodily tissues, including the bones, whereas its sister, magnesium, exerts a relaxing effect. In fact, calcium and magnesium work together to ensure proper muscle contraction and relaxation as well as the building of muscle fibers and connective tissues. Calcium also builds and maintains strong bones and teeth, is involved in the regulation of heart rhythm, aids the passage of nutrients into cell walls, assists in normal blood clotting, helps maintain normal blood pressure and is essential to normal kidney function.

A deficiency in calcium is common and can be signaled by muscle cramps; tingling in the lips, fingers and feet; leg numbness; tooth decay; sensitivity to noise; depression and deterioration of the bones (osteoporosis). Too much calcium, however, is known to be implicated in bone brittleness, whereas sufficient magnesium intake will allow the bones the necessary "give" to counteract jarring and sudden impacts.

Fibromyalgia-friendly food sources high in calcium are dried peas, canned sardines and salmon (including the bones), oranges, nuts, seeds, root vegetables and leafy green vegetables. As a low dairy diet is advisable for people with fibromyalgia, a magnesium/calcium/zinc supplement should make up the shortfall.

The RDA is 800 mg. However, the RDA for fibromyalgia is 1000 mg.

Magnesium

This important mineral aids the absorption of calcium, phosphorus, potassium, vitamins C and E, and the B complex vitamins. It is integral to the regulation and maintenance of normal heart activity; it helps to make bones less prone to breakage, and, together with calcium and vitamin C, aids the conversion of blood sugar into energy.

Magnesium deficiency is as common as that of calcium and, due to the precarious balance between these two associated minerals, deficiency can also be caused by excessive calcium supplementation. Junk foods are frequently low in magnesium, and processed bran added to a poor diet can render magnesium useless. Deficiency symptoms include muscle pain and tenderness, fatigue, migraine and headaches, tremor and shakiness, poor mental function, allergies, palpitations and numbness and tingling in the fingers and toes.

As it appears that all fibromyalgics suffer magnesium deficiencies, supplementation is highly recommended.

Fibromyalgia-friendly food sources high in magnesium include whole grains, leafy green vegetables, nuts—especially almonds and cashews—seeds, legumes, tofu and soy products and vegetables—especially broccoli, sweet corn, bananas and apricots.

The RDA is 270 mg. However, the RDA for fibromyalgia is 600 mg.

Manganese

Part of an important antioxidant enzyme system, manganese plays a vital role in fibromyalgia. It helps create energy from glucose and aids in the normalization of the central nervous system. It is also essential for normal skeletal development; activates enzymes known to be helpful in the digestion and utilization of foods, and plays a key role in the breakdown of fats and cholesterol.

Deficiency symptoms include digestive problems, dizziness, paralysis and convulsions.

Fibromyalgia-friendly food sources high in manganese are leafy green vegetables, whole grains, nuts, seeds and tea.

The RDA for fibromyalgia is 10 mg.

Zinc

Another important antioxidant, zinc is involved in blood stability; wound-healing; protein synthesis, digestion and the development and maintenance of the reproductive organs. This mineral is often low in Western diets. Vegetarian diets may be especially deficient—the high grain content binds the zinc, rendering it useless. This mineral is also crucial to growth and development; hair and nail growth; the formation of skin and insulin output.

Zinc should be accompanied by copper in a ratio of 10–15 mg of zinc to 1 mg of copper, to prevent a possible copper imbalance.

Deficiency symptoms include white spots on the finger nails, stretch marks, fatigue, decreased alertness, susceptibility to infections and delayed sexual maturity.

Fibromyalgia-friendly food sources high in zinc are the herb licorice, oysters, lean meats, liver, wheat germ, pumpkin seeds, sunflower seeds and ginseng.

The RDA is 15 mg and fibromyalgics require approximately this amount.

Selenium

A major antioxidant, this mineral protects cells from the toxic effects of free radicals and, in so doing, boosts the immune system. In the process of oxidation, selenium slows down the aging and hardening of tissues and preserves tissue elasticity. It is also beneficial for the prevention and treatment of dandruff.

Selenium deficiency symptoms include premature aging, loose skin, dandruff and heart disease.

Fibromyalgia-friendly food sources high in selenium are tuna, salmon, shrimps, garlic, tomatoes, sunflower seeds, Brazil nuts and wheat breads.

The RDA for fibromyalgia is 100 mcg.

Potassium

This mineral works with sodium to regulate heart and muscle function. It also ensures the normal transmission of nerve impulses; aids normal growth; stimulates the kidneys to eliminate toxic body waste; and promotes healthy skin.

Deficiency symptoms include poor reflexes, muscle twitches, weakness and soreness, nervous disorders, erratic and/or rapid heartbeats, insomnia, fatigue and high cholesterol levels.

Fibromyalgia-friendly food sources high in potassium are bananas, lean meats, avocados, tomato juice, fruit juice, nuts, salad vegetables, potatoes, oranges and dried fruits.

The RDA is 3500 mg. However, the RDA for fibromyalgia is 5000 mg.

Chromium

Chromium is part of what is known as the "glucose tolerance factor," which means that it helps the body to metabolize sugar and stabilize blood sugar levels. It also increases the efficiency of insulin in metabolizing carbohydrates.

Chromium deficiency is indicated by weight loss, glucose intolerance, tiredness, diabetes and heart disease.

Fibromyalgia-friendly food sources high in chromium are brewer's yeast, mushrooms, wheat germ and low-fat cheese.

The RDA is 200 mcg.

Other Useful Supplements

Malic acid

Essential for energy production, malic acid is of prime importance in the treatment of fibromyalgia. It is also vital for reducing the toxic effects of aluminum—a scourge in autoimmune diseases such as fibromyalgia.

When combined with magnesium, malic acid can be particularly effective, so some supplement manufacturers now offer "magnesium malate," which combines the two.

Fibromyalgia-friendly food sources high in malic acid are all fruits, but apples have by far the highest content.

The RDA for fibromyalgia is 200 mg.

5-Hydroxytryptophan (5-HTP)

Because of its ability to increase serotonin levels, this phytonutrient (plant derivative) is known to be useful for treating fibromyalgia. Its benefits include pain, anxiety and fatigue reduction. It is also known to improve sleep.

The RDA for fibromyalgics is 100–500 mg daily, depending on the individual (see also Chapter 3). As with all other supplements, please consult your doctor before starting 5-HTP supplementation.

Glucosamine

A type of nutrient known as an "amino sugar," glucosamine governs the number of water-holding molecules in cartilage and is converted to larger molecules that make up connective tissue. This nutrient is now known to be effective in reducing the effects of arthritic conditions. In a study known as the Vulvodynia Project, led by Dr. C. C. Solomons in Denver, Colorado, in 1997, it successfully decreased pain and sensitivity in the soft tissues (muscles, ligaments and tendons) of subjects with fibromyalgia.

Available only as a nutritional supplement, it is often combined with vitamin C and the amino acid tyrosine to maximize its action.

The RDA for fibromyalgia is 1000 mg.

Boron

This trace element is important in maintaining good muscular health. It is also believed to reduce calcium loss in postmenopausal women.

Deficiency symptoms are thought to include osteoporosis and menopausal symptoms in women.

Fibromyalgia-friendly food sources high in boron are apples, pears, prunes, seeds, raisins, tomatoes and cauliflower.

The RDA for fibromyalgia is 3 mg.

Co-enzyme Q10

This enzyme aids the transfer of oxygen and energy between components of the cells and between the blood and the tissues. It is highly beneficial to people with nutritional deficiencies, such as fibromyalgia sufferers.

Fibromyalgia-friendly food sources high in Co-enzyme Q10 are peanuts and other nuts, mackerel, chicken, whole grains, sardines and spinach.

Co-enzyme Q10 (also known as coQ10) can be purchased in capsule form from health food stores.

The RDA for fibromyalgics is 100 mg. Your doctor should be consulted before you begin co-enzyme Q10 supplementation.

DHEA (dehydroepiandosterone)

Secreted by the adrenal glands, DHEA is one of the most abundant hormones in the body. Its use has shown great benefits for immune system disorders such as fibromyalgia, osteoporosis and chronic fatigue syndrome. However, DHEA is produced naturally when good nutrition occurs. This hormone may only be obtained on prescription from your doctor.

Ginkgo biloba

The effectiveness of ginkgo biloba is now well documented. When used in the treatment of fibromyalgia, this herbal antioxidant can help maintain and support the body's circulation, particularly to the extremities—the hands and feet and, most importantly, the brain. The advantages include better cerebral blood flow; improved tissue oxygenation; more efficient energy production; and improved cognitive function—that is, concentration and short-term memory.

In two trials undertaken in the 1990s, volunteers were given ginkgo biloba daily. The first trial[13] showed that their short-term memories had improved significantly and, in the second,[14] the volunteers displayed even sharper reactions and better memories, as well as improved brain function—all of which were judged to be due to improved circulation. Ginkgo biloba is, therefore, considered very useful in the treatment of fibromyalgia.

This herb can be purchased in capsule form from health food stores, pharmacies and the larger supermarkets. The dosage instructions given on the label should be closely followed. As people on prescription medication—warfarin and aspirin—can react adversely to ginkgo biloba, please consult your doctor before taking this supplement.

Milk thistle

Milk thistle not only protects the liver from disease and damage due to ingested or inhaled toxins, it is also capable of regenerating damaged liver tissue. Unfortunately, though, milk thistle is ineffective when brewed into a tea.

Milk thistle can be purchased in capsule form and the label dosage instructions should be followed. Again, please consult your doctor before taking this herbal supplement.

Oil of evening primrose

This essential fatty acid of the omega 6 family is extracted from the seed of the evening primrose plant. It contains a percentage of gamma linolenic acid or GLA—a vital link in prostaglandin manufacture. (Prostaglandins are hormone-like substances involved in reducing inflammation in the body. They are also involved in blood clotting, blood pressure and hormone regulation.) However, conversion of linolenic acid (omega 6) to GLA can be slowed down by foods rich in saturated fat, alcohol, excessive sugar, zinc deficiency, stress and aging. When omega 6 conversion to GLA is inefficient, supplementation is highly recommended.

Oil of evening primrose is often taken by women prior to menstruation to help maintain GLA levels. Because it aids hormone balance, it is also recommended for people with fibromyalgia.

The RDA is 500–1000 mg.

Some Important Points to Remember About RDAs

In most instances, the recommended daily amounts (RDAs) of vitamin and mineral supplements set by the Department of Health are only intended to prevent common diseases associated with a severe deficiency. They are not intended to promote the optimal functioning and protection of bodily systems. RDAs, therefore, are the very minimum intake required for good health. For example, the RDA for vitamin E is 10 mg, but scientific research has shown that the level offering protection to the heart is in excess of 67 mg. Of course, this amount is inclusive of vitamin E obtained from natural sources.

The importance of a magnesium and malic acid combination

Supplements of magnesium and malic acid—also formulated as magnesium malate—are believed to markedly reduce the pain and fatigue of fibromyalgia.

As stated earlier, magnesium is essential to many bodily functions. However, it plays a vital role in the operation of the important malic acid shuttle service, which delivers vital nutrients to the cells. Malic acid enters the cycle at the most efficient site and is then converted into usable energy. As a component of what is known as the Kreb's cycle, malic acid also deals with the build-up of lactic acid in the muscles and other soft tissues.

In a study carried out in 1992,[15] volunteer fibromyalgics were given 6 to 12 tablets a day containing a magnesium and malic acid combination, each tablet consisting of 50 mg of magnesium and 200 mg of malic acid. After four weeks, their pain levels were halved. After another four weeks, they fell even more—from an initial pain score of 19.6, down to 6.5. For the next two weeks, six patients were then switched to a placebo (a sugar pill with no active ingredients, but the patients are not told this so they think they are taking medicine). Their pain scores rose from 6.5 to 21.5, the pain and fatigue distinctly worsening within 48 hours of switching to the placebo.

In a later study,[16] volunteer fibromyalgics were not informed whether they were taking the supplements or a placebo. The findings of the first study were confirmed, with the clarification that only patients taking at least six magnesium and malic acid combination supplements a day showed a significant reduction in pain.

Magnesium and malic acid appear to reduce the pain issuing from the "trigger points" found in fibromyalgia—these being specific sites from which pain radiates to other parts of the body.

To achieve the desired effect, you should take six 75-mg magnesium tablets a day (450 mg) for eight to 10 months to raise your levels to normal, then two tablets a day (150 mg) to maintain the improvement. A dose of 300 mg of malic acid—that is, 100 mg, taken three times a day—should be followed initially, dropping to a maintenance level of 100 mg daily after eight to 10 months.

Magnesium and malic acid supplements may be bought separately or else combined in the form of magnesium malate. However, you would be advised to consult your doctor before embarking on this treatment. Diarrhea is a possible side effect.

Guidance on Taking Supplements

Studies have shown that vitamins A, C and E (known as the "ACE" vitamins), together with co-enzyme Q10, selenium, zinc and manganese supplements, work as fine antioxidants, reducing the oxidative stress of fibromyalgia and aiding the healing process. These substances may be purchased together in a single antioxidant supplement from certain health supplement manufacturers, and are sold under different brand names. Alternatively the constituents may be bought separately, but generally at a higher price. Trials have shown that the above-mentioned combination of supplements should be taken for a period of one month before commencing further radical supplementation. However, evening primrose oil and B complex supplementation could be started after two weeks. Remember that it is important to take sufficient vitamin B_5 (pantothenic acid).

During month two, I would suggest that you begin magnesium and malic acid supplementation. A multimineral supplement containing calcium, manganese, zinc, boron and magnesium should also be taken.

During months three and four, it would be helpful to begin taking 5-HTP, together with ginkgo biloba, co-enzyme Q10, glucosamine and milk thistle. All of these work in different ways to improve the symptoms of fibromyalgia.

I appreciate that a fair amount of expenditure is called for to do this, but, because of the many deficiencies in fibromyalgia, supplementation is very important. Apart from following a healthy diet, there is, to date, no better way to significantly reduce your symptoms. By following the diet alone, you should make a noticeable difference to your health, but, by incorporating the recommended supplements into your regime, you will give your body an even greater chance of healing. Having said that, please remember that to take only one or two types of supplements is better than taking none at all. The antioxidant supplements are of prime importance, as is the magnesium and malic acid (magnesium malate) supplement.

As we are all very different, I would advise that you test the effects of each supplement to assess the required dosage for you, maybe even commencing each type of supplement separately to more accurately judge its effects. You may actually require a higher or lower dosage than initially supposed. High levels should, however, be reduced to maintenance levels after eight to 10 months.

Because there is some doubt as to the amounts of certain supplements needed to treat fibromyalgia, you may prefer to consult a nutritionist. He or she will not only advise you about correct dosages but also give clear and careful guidance regarding your diet.

11

Substances to Avoid

Although I have already outlined the dangers of chemically grown produce and toxic food additives, there are, unfortunately, many more inhospitable foods and substances that ultimately suppress our immune systems and cause other damage. People with fibromyalgia are particularly susceptible to the effects of such substances.

Stimulants

Our bodies need rest and relaxation in order to function at optimum levels. When these are withheld, high stress levels make us crave stimulants to help us continue to function. Alcohol, cigarettes, caffeine-containing products, such as coffee, tea, cocoa and chocolate, and products containing refined white sugar, such as cakes, cookies and sweets, provide an energy "lift." They stimulate our systems. Unfortunately, not only is the lift short-lived, leaving us feeling lower than before in its wake, these substances are also known to be detrimental to our health.

The elimination of stimulants should bring about improvements in every area in fibromyalgia—particularly where energy levels and anxiety are concerned. If you find that you are unable to completely eliminate stimulants from your diet, however, reduce them as much as possible—it will make a difference.

In general, you may find this diet easier to adhere to if you allow yourself an occasional treat. Try to beware of letting treats become routine, however! Obviously the strategy for smoking is different. If you manage to cut out smoking, an occasional cigarette will risk undoing all your hard work.

Caffeine

Caffeine products can not only cause stress to the adrenal glands, they are also toxic to the liver. In addition they can also reduce the body's ability to absorb vitamins and minerals. Caffeine is addictive, too—it has cocaine, morphine, strychnine, nicotine and atropine as close family members, and all of these are nerve poisons. Consumed regularly, coffee and other caffeine-containing products, such as tea, chocolate, cocoa and cola drinks, are also likely to give rise to chronic anxiety, the symptoms of which are agitation, palpitations, headaches, indigestion, panic, insomnia and hyperventilation. Chronic anxiety is a symptom commonly occurring with fibromyalgia. However, it is the toxicity of caffeine that may contribute to the development of fibromyalgia. My best advice is to remove caffeine products from your diet.

Unfortunately, because caffeine is addictive, reducing intake is far from easy. Withdrawal symptoms can take the form of splitting headaches, fatigue, depression, poor concentration and muscle pains. It is no wonder people can feel terrible until they have had their first dose of caffeine in the morning and that they cannot seem to function properly without regular doses throughout the day!

Caffeine is "washed out" of the system very quickly, however, so it is possible to minimize withdrawal symptoms by gradually reducing your intake over several weeks. Believe me, when it has been totally removed from your system, you certainly feel the difference!

Sugar

It has been said that after stress, alcohol and drugs, sugar poses the greatest risk to health in the Western world. It is added to almost all processed and pre-prepared foods and has a drug-like effect on the body. A couple of cookies or a slice of cake will provide us with an instant lift, but to the detriment of our long-term health. Sugar fills us up in place of the foods our bodies need. Furthermore, it has no nutritional value, providing us with empty calories that only cause us to put on weight via insulin, the fat-storage hormone.

Stone Age people only had access to the unrefined sugars present in fruit—"unrefined" meaning not having undergone any form of processing. The only refined sugar available to them was honey, but their digestive systems were able to handle this occasional excess. Nowadays, many refined sugars are available to us, but, unfortunately, our bodies have not progressed enough to enable us to cope with them efficiently.

It does not help that modern people have trained themselves to have a sweet tooth. There are alternatives to sugar, however. For example, you can sweeten your drinks and desserts by adding fresh fruit, or baked apples by sprinkling on cinnamon.

Here are some alternatives to refined white sugar.

- **Honey**   Raw, unprocessed honey is high in enzymes. Half a cup of honey replaces one cup of refined white sugar.
- **Fructose**   The sugar from fruit resembles white table sugar but, like sugar, it is of no nutritional value. As it requires processing by the liver, it should be used in moderation. Half a cup of fructose replaces one cup of refined white sugar.
- **Muscovado or turbinado**   Muscovado sugar is the first crude crystals that appear when sugar beet and cane are processed. It is brown and sticky and contains healthy organic acids. One cup of muscovado replaces one cup of refined white sugar.
- **Molasses**   The residue from the first stage of crystalization from sugar beet and cane is molasses, which is bitter and black. Like muscovado, it, too, is rich in organic acids. Half a cup of molasses replaces one cup of refined white sugar.
- **Demerara sugar or soft brown sugar or Barbados sugar**   This comes from the next stage of the sugar refining process. As it has still undergone far less processing than ordinary white sugar, it contains more nutrients, including organic acids. One cup of demerara or soft brown sugar replaces one cup of refined white sugar.
- **Brown rice syrup**   The slow boiling of brown rice results in a thick, honey-like syrup. One cup of brown rice syrup replaces one cup of refined white sugar.

- **Date sugar** Made from ground, dehydrated dates, date sugar has a high vitamin and mineral content. Two-thirds of a cup of date sugar replaces one cup of refined white sugar.
- **Barley malt** A syrup made from roasted barley, barley malt contains several minerals and trace amounts of the B vitamins. One cup of barley malt replaces one cup of refined white sugar.
- **Fruit juice sweetener** This is simply unprocessed fruit juice, offering all the vitamins and minerals of fruit. One cup of this sweetener replaces one cup of refined white sugar.
- **Maple syrup** Made from boiled down maple tree sap, half a cup of maple syrup replaces one cup of refined white sugar.

All the above-mentioned white sugar substitutes may be used in cooking and baking.

Alcohol

As fibromyalgia is a disorder of the central nervous system and alcohol is a nerve poison, consuming alcohol can further complicate the nerve transmission process. It may work well as an analgesic, but the effects are short-lived.

Alcohol consumption is known to deplete the B vitamins and probably antioxidants as they are required to mop up the damaging free radicals stimulated by the liver's alcohol detoxification process. In the long term, anything but very modest alcohol consumption is likely to cause more problems than it takes away. I would recommend, therefore, that it be consumed in moderation, if at all.

Even more damaging is the fact that pesticides, colorants and other harmful additives are generally involved in modern-day alcohol production, exerting further strain on the liver. If you cannot avoid the occasional drink, red wine would appear to be the best choice.

Tobacco

Cigarette and cigar smoking increases the number of destructive free radicals within the body. In addition, smokers have low levels of selenium and vitamins A, C and E—all of which are active antioxidants. Smokers also carry high levels of cadmium, a toxic metal, in their bodies. My best advice is to give up smoking.

Aspartame

Aspartame, a widely used artificial sweetener, is surrounded by controversy. When given to monkeys in tests it proved harmless, but that, it is now believed, is because of the highly nutritious, antioxidant-rich foods these animals consume. Experts have now drawn the conclusion that aspartame is harmless to individuals on antioxidant-rich diets but may cause problems in people who are not.

I have now read several articles about the unwelcome side effects of aspartame and conclude that perhaps we fibromyalgics should err on the side of caution. "Aspartame poisoning" is said to produce many of the symptoms and conditions occurring in fibromyalgia. These include muscle spasms, shooting pains, joint pain, depression, anxiety, fatigue and weakness, headaches, sleep problems, dizziness, diarrhea, tinnitus, mood changes, blurred vision and short-term memory loss.

Nancy Markle, an expert on multiple sclerosis, stated at a recent World Environment Conference that aspartame can be dangerous to diabetics, multiple sclerosis patients and people with Parkinson's disease. Neurosurgeon Dr. Russell Blakelock states in his book *Excitotoxins: The Taste That Kills* (Health Press Books, 1996) that the ingredients of aspartame can overstimulate the neurons of the brain, giving rise to dangerous symptoms. Dr. H. J. Roberts, a diabetic specialist, has written a book entitled *Defense Against Alzheimer's Disease* (Sunshine Sentinel Press Inc., 1995) in which he states that aspartame poisoning is escalating the incidence of Alzheimer's disease.

In a recent article, Nancy Markle writes that there were speakers and ambassadors from different nations at the World Environment Conference who promised to help spread the word. She added that there is actually no reason to use aspartame and that it is not, in effect, a diet product. In fact, the congressional record states: "It [aspartame] causes a craving for carbohydrates and will cause weight gain." One doctor revealed that when he got people to stop their intake of aspartame, their average weight loss was 19 pounds per person.

If the label says "sugar free" or "diet," I would advise you to check the list of additives. The brand-name aspartame products should be avoided, too.

Food Additives

Up to 80 percent of the foods on our supermarket shelves have undergone some degree of refinement or chemical alteration.

Food additives to watch out for follow.

- **MSG** These letters stand for monosodium glutamate, which is the most common flavor enhancer on the market. It is often disguised as hydrolyzed yeast, autolyzed yeast, yeast extract, sodium caseinate, natural flavoring, vegetable protein, hydrolyzed protein, other spices, and natural chicken or turkey flavoring.
- **BHT** This is butylated hydroxyanisole, which is a widely used preservative. It is used in baked goods, breakfast cereals, potatoes, pastry mixes, dry mixes for desserts, chewing gum, sweets, ice cream and so on. BHT can adversely affect liver and kidney function and has been associated with behavioral problems in children.
- **Sorbate** A preservative and fungus preventative, sorbate can be found in drinks, baked goods, pie fillings, artificially sweetened jellies, preserves, prepared salads and fresh fruit cocktails.
- **Sulphites** Used in bleaching and preserving certain foods, this substance prevents the discoloration of light-colored fruit and vegetables, enabling them to look fresh for longer. Sulphites are often found in beer, lager, wine and sliced fruit. They may also be present in packaged wine vinegar, gravies, avocado dip, sauces, potatoes and lemon juice.
- **Aspartame** Mentioned earlier in this chapter, aspartame has been linked with problems in many systems in the body. It is often found in foods described as "low sugar," "sugar free," or "diet."

Junk Food

It is a fact that chemically "enhanced" foods sap our energy resources. The body uses a great deal of energy in the digestion, absorption, cleansing and elimination of foods. It uses far more energy in striving to metabolize low-quality foods, which, unfortunately, hold little nutritional value.

In fibromyalgia particularly, the body is unable to find sufficient energy to complete the digestive process efficiently. As a result, toxins and debris can be stored in the body. Unfortunately, toxic buildup affects every part of the body, from the neurons of the brain to the arteries, kidneys and liver.

Water

There is much ongoing discussion as to the suitability of tap water for human consumption. Water in the U.S. is thought to be superior to that of a number of other countries. However, it is still laden with toxic chemicals and inorganic salts that are detrimental to those with fibromyalgia.

In areas of "hard" water, where rainwater has run through limestone (containing sodium salts and calcium salts), our tap water has a high mineral content, particularly of mineral salts. Drinking such water can result in fluid retention and a concentration of salts in our tissues. Ultimately, it can even lead to high blood pressure and hardening of the arteries. "Soft" water, on the other hand, is usually filtered through sandstone and peat, which removes many of the impurities. This is better, until chemicals are added, such as chlorine and, in some areas, fluoride.

Our water is taken from the following sources:

- **Reservoirs** The aforementioned chemicals are added to this surface water.
- **Deep artesian wells** The purest source of water, artesian water is added to reservoirs;
- **Groundwater** A high content of suspended matter and dissolved acids give groundwater its brown color. Aluminum sulphate is added as a coagulant, then chemical polyelectrolytes are put in to further settle the coagulated waste. Although this water is then passed through sand filters to remove the settled particles, some of the chemicals remain in the water, which is then added to reservoir water.

As a result of the processes to which water is submitted, it can end up being saturated with inappropriate mineral salts and added chemicals. Other pollutants that often seep in then compound the situation.

As tap water is of some detriment to people with fibromyalgia, I recommend that purified water be used. The following types of water are recommended.

- **Distilled water**   Formed by boiling water and condensing the steam, distilled water is very pure. It successfully leaches excessive minerals and other salts from the body, but must only be used for periods of up to six months or else essential minerals are at risk of being removed as well. For maximum effect, not more than one of six or eight small glasses of distilled water must be consumed every hour. The results can be spectacular when used as an adjunct to the detoxification diet.
- **Filtered water**   Although distilled water has superior effects to filtered water during the detoxification diet, filtered water should be used to maintain your health. Water filters on the market vary from simple carbon filters to carbon filters with silver mesh components that even destroy bacteria. There are also reverse osmosis filters and these produce very clean water while still retaining some of the precious trace minerals. It must be said, however, that the individual effectiveness at removing pollutants is proportionate to their cost. Do not let this put you off, though. An inexpensive carbon filter is far better than no filter at all.

Note that distilled or filtered water should also be used to wash foods and make drinks.

Refined White Flours

Refined wheat flour is generally known to us as plain flour, but can also be called bread flour or pastry flour. In this instance, "refined" means that the husks have been removed and the remaining powder bleached. This results in the loss of its nutritional value—vitamins, minerals, protein and the fiber content all being removed by these processes. Only carbohydrates and calories remain.

Fortified flours have, as the name implies, had many of their nutrients replaced. However, vitamin B6 and folacin are not put back. Also, of the nine minerals initially removed, only three—iron, calcium and phosphorus—are returned. To compound the situation, many of the replaced processed nutrients have a very slow absorption rate when consumed. So, all in all, refined flours have little nutritional value.

Refined cornflour, or cornmeal, undergoes a less radical refinement process, so loses less of its nutritional content. The oils within the corn can turn rancid, however, if the "meal" is not freshly ground.

Healthy flour substitutes include whole grain, spelt, quinoa, oat, corn, brown rice, rye, barley, potato and rice flours, all of which are rich in nutrients. Health food stores stock healthy bread mixes that are easy to prepare and nutritious.

Toxic Chemicals

Interestingly, apart from a few exceptions, it is no coincidence that in countries with little industrial power and where fresh food is eaten straight from the land, few people suffer chemical sensitivities, food intolerances and/or allergies.

Perhaps the most commonly contracted sensitivity is to "organophosphates," which are now widely used in farming throughout the Western world.

Organophosphates

Organophosphates (known as OPs) are extremely toxic chemicals used in crop production as a matter of course. It may surprise you to know that every system in the body can be adversely affected by OPs—particularly the immune system, which gives us antibody protection against disease, the central nervous system, which is the nerve processing center, and the endocrine system, which regulates hormone levels. All the aforementioned systems function abnormally in fibromyalgia.

Typical symptoms of OP poisoning include mental and physical fatigue, poor muscle stamina, muscle pain, drug intolerance, irritable bowel syndrome, sweating, low body temperature, numb patches, muscle twitching, clumsiness, mood swings, irritability, poor short-term memory and poor concentration. Many people with fibromyalgia display all these symptoms.

Evidence of OP poisoning can be found in the following ways.

- **Immune system**   Tests can show low levels of B cells, abnormal T suppressor/helper lymphocyte ratios, raised C reactive protein and other abnormalities.

- **Hormones**   Tests can show that the pituitary gland is suppressed. This will promote borderline thyroid activity, mild adrenal stress, low levels of sex hormones and low melatonin levels. As a result, the individual will suffer lethargy, weight gain, dry hair and skin, anxiety, low sex drive and sleep difficulties.
- **Cognitive function**   Psychometric tests can show impairment of short-term memory, the processing of information, concentration and the ability to learn.
- **Autonomic nervous system**   Nerve conduction testing can show abnormalities in many automatic functions. These include the body temperature, sweating, gut function, heart and respiratory rate, blood pressure and so on.
- **Liver function**   Tests can show slightly raised liver enzyme levels.
- **Blood count**   Tests can show low white cell count.
- **Trace element levels**   Tests can show deficiencies of magnesium.
- **Vitamins**   Tests can show deficiencies of the B vitamins.

Scary, isn't it? However, if you have fibromyalgia you can begin to eradicate these effects by consuming organically grown produce. The body can be aided in the detoxification of OPs by taking magnesium, selenium and vitamin B_{12} supplements.

Chemical Sensitivities

People who are sensitive to OPs may gradually become sensitive to other chemicals. This is known as the "spreading phenomenon." Multiple chemical sensitivities—sometimes referred to as allergies—are common in fibromyalgia, sufferers often becoming sensitive to all manner of manmade products. They can react adversely to perfumes, cigarette smoke, alcohol, pesticides, artificial fertilizers, petrochemical fumes, glue, varnish, aerosol sprays, some carpets, some cosmetics, some household cleaners, some paints, etc.

Sensitization to chronic chemical exposure is now well documented. Mechanics can become sensitized to gasoline fumes, painters to paint, printers to ink, and so on. Maybe we should all take a closer look at our immediate environments.

The body's tolerance of chemicals can be raised, however, by following the fibromyalgia healing diet, taking plenty of rest and relaxation and adhering to a regular, gentle exercise regime.

Heavy metals

You may be surprised to learn that our bodies commonly absorb heavy metals that are toxic to our systems. The following are the chief culprits.

ALUMINUM

Believed to be highly implicated in the evolution and persistence of fibromyalgia, high levels of aluminum are harmful to the central nervous system.

Sources of aluminum poisoning may be foil, cookware, containers and underarm deodorants. This metal can also be found in coffee, bleached white flour and antacid medications.

Interestingly, experts are now of the opinion that magnesium and calcium deficiencies increase the toxic effects of ingested aluminum.

MERCURY

Those of us with amalgam tooth fillings are ingesting minute amounts of mercury vapor every day—and mercury is the second most toxic heavy metal in the world. The leaked mercury vapor confuses the immune system into attacking the body's own tissues, including the muscles, tendons and ligaments. For this reason, mercury fillings are thought to be implicated in the onset of fibromyalgia.

As a result of mercury intake, the immune system also sets up antibodies against certain foods, thus causing the many food intolerances we see in fibromyalgia. Synthetic white fillings may be a safe alternative.

LEAD

Ingestion of this metal is known to cause neurological and psychological disturbance. Some old houses still have lead piping, through which the drinking water is carried, while others have copper piping fused together with lead-based solder. The use of a water filter is highly recommended in such cases, although, obviously, to have the piping replaced by modern copper or synthetic piping is the ideal.

I would like to reinforce my earlier point that fruits and vegetables should be washed in filtered water before use to help remove unwanted substances. A tablespoonful of vinegar may be added to the water to aid this process.

CADMIUM

High carbohydrate consumption is linked with high cadmium levels in the body. Cigarette smoking is another cause of cadmium buildup—cadmium being mainly absorbed via the lungs. This metal is known to be damaging to the kidneys and lungs. It can, however, be gradually removed by a detoxification diet, followed by good nutrition.

12

The Detoxification Program

Large amounts of pesticides, food additives and preservatives, toxic chemicals, heavy metals and stimulants can be stored in our organs and tissues, perpetuating fibromyalgia and laying us open to further disease. Although only small amounts of pollutants are ingested each day, over many years—even decades—it can result in toxic overload, some experts estimating that certain adults carry pounds of toxic byproducts and waste. These experts believe that we consume approximately one gallon of pesticides (found on fresh foods) and 11½ pounds of chemical food additives a year.

The detoxification process gives the body a well-earned rest, allowing it to concentrate on eliminating toxins and regenerating damaged tissues. Detoxification ensures that toxic byproducts and waste are pulled from the cells into the bloodstream, from where they reach the liver and kidneys, the organs of detoxification. These two organs then work to eliminate the toxins from the body.

Cleansing will only occur, however, if we provide our bodies with cleansing fuel. Fruits, vegetables, juices and water are perfect for this process as they require minimal digestion. The energy saved is then utilized for the elimination of toxins and debris. Secondary to these are whole grains and cereals, oils, nuts, seeds, herbs and spices. They are not only useful in detoxification but also contain important nutrients and use minimum energy during their digestion and elimination.

Nutritionists recommend a 21-day detoxification program for people with fibromyalgia, after which an improved diet, the type of which is described in this book, should be followed. However, I recommend that you read this chapter before commencing the detoxification program.

Retraining Your Palate

The fibromyalgia healing diet and detoxification program require that you retrain your palate to accept foods in their more natural form. People who have eaten a lot of sugar, salt and saturated fats (those that are solid at room temperature) have come to expect those particular tastes. I recommend, therefore, that, before embarking on the detoxification program, you cut back gradually on the amounts of sugar, salt and fat you consume. At the same time, try to slowly replace products made from white refined flour with products made from whole-grain flours and use only whole-grain flours in cooking and baking.

The following steps are recommended as part of such a gradual change.

- Eat one cookie instead of two and slice yourself a smaller piece of cake prior to cutting out or minimizing foods made with butter, sugar and white refined flour.
- To get extra vitamins and minerals, add chopped, cooked vegetables to a can of soup before cutting out or minimizing use of canned products.
- Reduce your intake of caffeine products very gradually. Withdrawing too fast may cause fatigue and headaches. If possible, remove caffeine from your diet before commencing the detoxification program.
- Get into the habit of snacking on a variety of nuts, such as almonds, cashews, Brazils and pecans, dried fruit, such as raisins, dates and apricots, and seeds, such as pumpkin, sesame, sunflower and flaxseeds.
- Select a salad or vegetables instead of fries when eating out.
- Get into the habit of drinking fruit juice instead of carbonated drinks, which affect carbon levels within the body. Fruit juices generally satisfy a sweet tooth and can be diluted with water so they go further.

- Slowly increase the number and variety of fruits and vegetables you use.
- Gradually reduce the amount of salt you add to your food and in cooking, using rock or sea salt in place of table salt.
- If you find you are craving sugar, remember that the lift it offers will be very temporary—the next effect being a plummet into a low mood. Staving off hunger with fruit (fresh and dried), nuts and seeds is not only a far healthier choice, it also stabilizes blood-sugar levels, helping to ward off the low mood.
- Wash fruit and vegetables thoroughly before use, adding a little vinegar to the distilled or filtered water you use. If you do buy produce that is not organically grown, remember that it will probably have been sprayed with pesticides.

I will just add that, in adulthood, we often do things we do not particularly enjoy. We do them, however, because it is the right thing to do. Cutting down on pleasant foods can be difficult, but our cravings for these foods really can disappear, given a little time and determination.

I must mention also that the people who follow this diet generally admit to finding it enjoyable after the first few weeks. There is no need to become obsessive about it, though! Any improvement in your diet will benefit your condition.

The Detoxification Superfoods

Here you will find lists of the foods that are known to be powerful detoxifiers. If possible, your detoxification program should mainly consist of the following.

Fruit

Try to make fruit a staple of your detoxification program. Not only is it packed with vitamins, minerals, amino acids and enzymes, but its high fiber content means that it is a perfect internal cleanser, too. The fiber binds with toxins and the water content of fruit helps to flush them out. In addition, the pectin in fruit is known to bind with certain heavy metals, helping to carry them from the body.

- **Lemons** During detoxification, try to start your day with a glass of hot water with freshly squeezed lemon juice. As well as providing vitamin C, lemon juice stimulates the liver and gall bladder. It is a powerful cleanser and antiseptic.

- **Apples**   Containing malic and tartaric acid, apples boost digestion and aid the removal of impurities from the liver. Their high fiber and pectin content also ensure that they help to eliminate toxins and purify the system. Apples are rich in vitamin C and beta-carotene.
- **Oranges**   This fruit stimulates digestion and, as well as containing high levels of vitamin C and other nutrients, is a powerful antioxidant.
- **Grapefruit**   Grapefruit is not only high in vitamin C, beta-carotene, calcium, phosphorus and potassium but also stimulates digestion.
- **Pears**   Because of their high water content, pears are a diuretic, stimulating the removal of excess water from the body. They contain vitamin C, fiber, potassium and pectin.
- **Bananas**   Containing fiber, vitamins and potassium, bananas provide plenty of energy, making them useful during detoxification.
- **Grapes**   This fruit is one of the most effective detoxifiers. Grapes are beneficial, too, for disorders of the liver, kidneys, digestion and skin. As they are often sprayed liberally with pesticides, though, it is important to wash them thoroughly or buy organic ones.
- **Melons**   Because of their high water content, melons are diuretics, aiding the removal of any excess fluid from the body. They contain vitamin C and beta-carotene.
- **Pineapples**   This fruit contains bromelain—an antibacterial agent that aids the digestion of protein. It also has anti-inflammatory properties.
- **Cherries**   Containing vitamin C, B vitamins and potassium, cherries assist the removal of toxins from the liver, kidneys and digestive system. The darker the cherry, the more effective it will be.
- **Mangoes**   Rich in vitamin C, beta-carotene and potassium, mangoes can cleanse the blood. For this reason, they are of great benefit during the detoxification program.

As dried fruit is a good source of nutrients, it is also a useful detoxifier. Fruit juices have great benefits, too, as they are so easy to digest. In addition, they help to speed up the metabolism, improve energy levels and stimulate the cleansing process.

Vegetables

Like fruit, vegetables should be a mainstay of a detoxification program. Vegetables are full of vitamins, minerals, bioflavonoids and plant nutrients (phytochemicals). They also exert a calming effect on the body.

- **Carrots** These vegetables are believed to cleanse, nourish and stimulate the whole body, particularly the kidneys, liver and digestive system. Fresh carrot juice offers the best benefits.
- **Onions, garlic and leeks** With their excellent antiviral and antibacterial nutrients, these vegetables are said to cleanse the whole system. Garlic boosts the immune system and has anti-inflammatory properties.
- **Broccoli, cabbage, cauliflower, Brussels sprouts, watercress and rutabaga** Members of the "cruciferous" family, these vegetables not only stimulate the liver but also stimulate the body's enzyme defenses, thereby playing a vital role in fighting disease.
- **Spinach** This vegetable is rich in beta-carotene and vitamin C. It also contains many more important antioxidant nutrients and is an excellent aid to detoxification.
- **Tomatoes** Containing many vital nutrients, tomatoes are said to stimulate the liver and so aid the removal of toxins.
- **Celery** This vegetable helps to remove excess fluid from the body.
- **Cucumber** Also a diuretic, cucumber aids digestion and relaxes the system.
- **Lettuce** Containing vitamin C, beta-carotene, folate and iron, lettuce has calming, sedative properties. The darker the leaf, the more nutritious it is.

Grains

Because whole grains and cereals are excellent sources of protein, complex carbohydrates, fiber, vitamins and minerals, they play a vital role in a detoxification program. Look for grains that are largely unprocessed as their high fiber content will speed up the passage of food through the bowel. Examples are brown rice, couscous, millet, barley, bulgar wheat, whole wheat, oats, barley, rye, corn, spelt, quinoa and buckwheat.

Beans and legumes

Similarly, the high fiber content of beans and legumes such as lentils, soy beans, chickpeas and dried peas makes them an important component of the detoxification program. They are also highly nutritious.

If you are unable to find organic beans that are canned in water, dried beans are a good alternative. However, most dried beans require soaking for at least eight hours prior to cooking. The preparation instructions should then be carefully followed, especially for kidney beans; otherwise they can be harmful.

Nuts and seeds

Nuts and seeds support the immune system during the detoxification process. They are also excellent sources of nutrients and oils. However, they are high in fat and should be eaten in moderation. Salted, coated nuts should be avoided.

Oils and vinegars

Although unsaturated oils (fat)—those that are liquid at room temperature—are an important part of a detoxification program, saturated fat should be avoided. Oils such as extra virgin olive oil and cold-pressed oils such as safflower, sunflower and canola oils provide essential fatty acids as well as vitamin E.

Organic apple cider vinegar stimulates digestion and has many health-giving properties. Other vinegars are not recommended as they contain acetic acid, which hinders digestion.

Herbs

Valued for their therapeutic qualities, herbs can be useful during a detoxification program. The most beneficial include milk thistle, echinacea, ginger root, gotu kola, goldenseal and dandelion leaf and root. Herbal tea infusions are nourishing and cleansing, too.

Spices

Spices have a cleansing, antiseptic effect on the body. Fresh ginger root is a powerful healing spice, as are cardamom, cinnamon, coriander, turmeric, nutmeg and fenugreek.

Dairy products

Dairy products are mucus-forming, and mucus will not only be present in the nasal and respiratory passages, it can also lurk in virtually every part of the body. In the bowel, mucus slows the transport of waste material, hampering the elimination of toxins and debris. Alternative foods include soy milk, rice milk, goats' milk and cheese, and tofu yogurts. The only divergence during detoxification should be butter, which must be spread very thinly on your whole-grain breads and rye crispbreads, and natural live yogurt.

Natural live yogurt

Try to eat a helping of natural live yogurt every day to improve the condition of your intestinal flora during detoxification. Natural live yogurt contains beneficial bacteria that rebalance the later flora.

Keeping a Diary

Keeping a food intake diary is an excellent way to monitor your progress. Seeing for yourself where you are making mistakes will ensure a smoother changeover to healthier eating.

Goals

It is a good idea to set goals at the start of the diary. For example, you may want to make a goal of eating two types of vegetables every day. Without the diary, you may assume you have done badly, but, on reading your entries, you may see that you have actually eaten two types of vegetables three or four times a week. That is a good starting point. Now you can focus on slowly increasing that amount. (Remember that it is important to become accustomed to the new foods in your diet before commencing the detoxification program.)

Here are some examples of goals toward maximum healing:

- eat two to three types of vegetables every day;
- eat two to three portions of fruit every day;
- cut out caffeine—coffee, chocolate, cola drinks, cocoa;
- cut out junk food;
- cut out table sugar and other sugar-containing products, such as cakes, candy, cookies, sugar-coated cereals and so on;
- cut out saturated fats;
- cut out refined white flour;
- eat only "whole" foods—whole wheat, corn, barley, brown rice and so on;
- drink eight to 10 glasses of clean water daily, including that in fruit juices and herbal teas;
- cut out or minimize table salt sprinkled on food, using small amounts of sea or rock salt instead;
- minimize the amount of salt added to cooking and baking;
- reduce your intake of meat and dairy products to a minimum, making sure to spread butter thinly (meat and dairy products should, ideally, be avoided for the duration of the detoxification program);
- minimize alcohol consumption;
- eat nuts, seeds and/or dried fruit as snacks once or twice a day;
- cut out artificial sweeteners;
- always check food labels for additives, preservatives and so on;
- buy only organically grown produce;
- use vegetable, corn or olive oil in cooking and dressings—extra virgin olive oil is best;
- cut out fried foods.

Note that if you are unable to entirely eliminate certain foods, you should not feel discouraged. Cutting down your intake will reduce the strain on your digestive system and detoxification organs, making a difference to your health.

A symptom column

It is also important to include a symptom column at the end of each month. It should include average energy levels, pain levels, headaches/migraines, muscle cramps, stiffness, aching joints, mood, sleep quality, stomach problems, cold hands and feet, general tiredness, concentration, short-term memory and stress levels. Each entry should be marked on a scale of one to ten, with the lowest numbers being the least intensity and higher numbers being greater intensity. This should show improvements that may otherwise be overlooked.

Weight Matters

It is no wonder that many people with fibromyalgia are overweight. Fibromyalgia demands that we are fairly inactive, cell energy production is limited and our metabolisms are sluggish.

As you well know, being overweight can be damaging to health. Its related conditions include high blood pressure, heart disease, diabetes, chronic anxiety and depression. However, it is not wise to lose weight by following either a crash diet or a diet that limits certain foods. Such diets almost certainly result in substantial weight loss in the early weeks, but the long-term result is actually weight gain. This occurs because the body goes into starvation mode, storing energy as fat in the cell pockets. Unfortunately, when the diet peters out, the weight piles on.

However, a positive side effect of a detoxification program, followed by a good-quality diet, is weight loss in people who are overweight. Furthermore, because the foods used are low in calories, any excess fat comes away—and with it all the toxins stored there!

A Healing Crisis

It is not all roses, however. A detoxification diet releases toxins and debris into the bloodstream, where they circulate until reaching the liver and kidneys. These organs then neutralize the toxins and prepare them for elimination. When the quantity of toxins exceeds the body's ability to remove them, though, detoxification reactions can occur. Toxins lingering in the bloodstream can cause lethargy, headaches and occasionally even diarrhea.

The good news is that the feeling of unwellness lasts for only a few days. Please do not let these possible side effects demotivate you for the ill feeling is a positive indication that the toxins are in the process of being removed. It is a sure sign that you are on your way to improved health. I must add that many people suffer no adverse reactions whatsoever.

Purified Water

During a detoxification program, distilled water is by far the most beneficial. It not only has cleansing properties but is also capable of drawing heavy metals, salts and other debris from the tissues. Drinking eight to 10 glasses of distilled water daily will considerably reduce detoxifying symptoms. After the detoxification program has been completed, you can return to filtered water.

If you are not able to obtain distilled water for your detoxification program, filtered water is an acceptable alternative. I would highly recommend that filtered water then be drunk for the rest of your life. However, if filtered water is not available, mineral water should be used. It is not the best choice, as it does not draw detrimental salts and so on from the tissues effectively, but is superior to tap water. Another method of "cleaning" your drinking water is to allow a jugful to stand in the freezer for a few hours before use. Remember to wash your fruit and vegetables in distilled or filtered or mineral water with a tablespoonful of vinegar added before eating or cooking.

Ready to Go!

Before getting started on the 21-day detoxification program, it is advisable to consciously tell yourself you are making an important lifestyle decision—to eat better. Remember that, as a result, your health will improve, the possibility of future illness will be reduced and you can look forward to a longer life!

The following guidelines should help you on your way to improved health:

- make optimum nutrition a goal—remind yourself of the importance of this goal to your health;
- make a conscious effort to change past bad eating behavior;
- be organized—plan meals in advance;
- eat three to five portions of fruit every day;
- eat three to five portions of vegetables every day, trying to occasionally eat raw vegetables, such as grated carrots with a salad;
- eat whole grains and cereals, nuts, beans, pulses, seeds, herbs, spices and the recommended oils;

- remember that fat must not be eliminated—consumption of unsaturated fat is essential for improved health;
- avoid skipping meals, particularly breakfast;
- boil, bake and steam your foods—eggs should be soft-boiled or poached;
- avoid overeating;
- do not ever go hungry;
- drink eight to 10 glasses of water a day, including that in fruit and vegetable drinks and herbal teas;
- if possible, try to keep busy to prevent boredom—this will help with any inclination you may feel toward eating to occupy time;
- avoid weighing and measuring yourself on a regular basis—instead, feel the benefit in the fit of your clothing;
- keep alcohol consumption very low, remembering that red wine is the best choice when you do have a drink;
- practice pain and stress management—daily deep breathing and relaxation exercises should cut stress levels and try to deal with negative thinking and irrational feelings by forward planning, being realistic and speaking openly of your limitations to others;
- follow a daily exercise program, expanding your routine and increasing the number of repetitions as you grow stronger, and ensure that you perform an aerobic activity—an exercise that makes you a little out of breath—at least once every other day;
- focus on getting well.

Your 21-day Detoxification Program

Just to reiterate, it is advisable to gradually accustom yourself to the different foods in your new diet. Giving yourself at least one month where you gradually introduce more and more of the recommended foods means that it is not such a shock to the system. This allows you time to get used to the tastes of newly introduced foods.

After a month—or longer if you wish—you can begin the 21-day detoxification program in earnest. The following are important points to remember:

- try to start your day with a glass of hot water with some freshly squeezed lemon juice added;

- eat a healthy breakfast, lunch and evening meal, but do not pile up the plate—if possible, consume 25 percent of your daily intake at breakfast, 50 percent at lunch and 25 percent in the evening, but, if you cannot manage this, don't worry, just make sure you do not eat too much toward the end of the day;
- eat regular snacks of fresh fruit, dried fruit, raw vegetables, nuts, seeds, crispbreads and so on (nuts and seeds—particularly cashew and pecan nuts, flaxseeds, sesame seeds and sunflower seeds—are excellent sources of essential oils and other important nutrients);
- increase your consumption of raw fruits, nuts, seeds and vegetables to at least 50 percent of your diet—"fruit and vegetables" should include apples, grapefruit, oranges, grapes, cherries, pineapple, avocados, melons, spinach, broccoli, Brussels sprouts, cabbage, lettuce, cucumber, radishes, onions, carrots and capsicum peppers;
- try to cut out all dairy products except natural live yogurt and butter, remembering to use only a small amount of the latter;
- eat whole grains and cereals, such as whole wheat, oats, barley, corn, couscous, millet, spelt and brown rice;
- eat beans, peas, lentils, herbs and spices;
- use olive, corn, safflower and sunflower oils;
- buy only organically grown produce—the superior taste makes up for the slight difference in cost;
- drink six to eight glasses of distilled or filtered water a day, making this up to the total of eight to 10 glasses of liquid recommended by drinking green tea and fruit and vegetable juices;
- have your last snack at least an hour before bedtime—eating a small amount of carbohydrate at the end of the day should encourage sleep;
- strive for a stress-free eating environment—no television or reading while eating;
- take exercise as tolerated;
- take in some fresh air every day;

- get plenty of rest, following a deep breathing and relaxation exercise at least once a day—you may want to use a relaxation tape to help you through the process and these can be purchased from health stores.

To achieve maximum detoxification, avoid or minimize your intake of the following:

- dairy products and meat—if you are unable to do this, eat only small, lean cuts in portions no larger or thicker than the size of your palm and remember that red meat in particular takes a long time to digest, using energy that could otherwise be utilized in detoxification;
- white refined sugar;
- white refined flour;
- additives and preservatives;
- foods grown using chemicals;
- junk food and salt;
- fried foods;
- caffeine, including coffee, caffeine teas, cola drinks, chocolate and cocoa;
- alcohol;
- tobacco;
- aspartame, saccharine and other refined or artificial sweeteners;
- finally, remember to take your drinks at least half an hour before and half an hour after eating—the greater the gap between eating and drinking, the less likelihood there is of important hydrochloric (stomach) acid being diluted.

Exercise and Fresh Air

Fundamental to the cleansing process is plenty of gentle, sustained exercise and daily fresh air. Exercise stimulates the lymph glands, which operate as a sewage system and, therefore, are heavily burdened during detoxification. The flow of lymph from the lymph glands is entirely dependent on muscular movement.

I know exercise is difficult for people with fibromyalgia, so keep it gentle. Circling your shoulders backward and forward several times a day will be beneficial, as will turning and tilting your head, full body side-dips and side-twists. Walking is good, too. You only need to walk around the house, maybe then climbing the stairs two or three times more than you would normally.

Having said that, fresh air is equally important as toxic gases are dispelled from our bodies via the lungs. The inhalation of clean, fresh oxygen sustains the metabolic reactions within each cell. You do not need to embark on a forced march every day, either! A walk around the garden once or twice a day or a short walk along the road should provide sufficient fresh air. If walking is difficult at this early stage, simply wrapping up warmly and standing at the open door or by an open window for a while is far better than nothing. Remember, too, that things will get better!

Nutrition Maintenance

You have successfully completed the detoxification program, so what happens now? Some of you may want to continue in the same vein. In the main, I would advise that you be a little less stringent, but try to eat the foods recommended in this book. Remember that, to continue the healing process, it is important to eat a wide variety of nutritious foods and take the recommended nutritional supplements. However, to maintain the detoxification of harmful chemicals and continue strengthening all the systems in the body, the following eating habits should be adhered to in the long term:

- continue to eat three or four small meals a day, remembering not to skip any;
- keep the high fiber content, eating fruits, vegetables, whole grains and cereals;
- have healthy food available at home or work so you can "snack" whenever you want;
- eat whole-grain breads, pasta and brown rice;
- eat plenty of legumes (peas and beans);
- select low-fat dairy products and keep your intake of them low;

- limit red meats, especially cured and smoked meats, as they are difficult to digest;
- eat white meats, tuna and fish in moderation;
- eat plenty of raw fruit and vegetables, making salads a must;
- consume at least eight glasses of liquid a day, including fruit/ vegetable juices and herbal teas.

It is important to remember that if you deviate from your diet—whether during detoxification or afterwards—do not be disheartened. Just return to your healthy foods and forget the slight lapse. There will be times when you prefer to put the diet aside for a while, such as when eating out or during a holiday. This does not mean that you have stopped your healthy diet. Take up where you left off as soon as you can and get back to improving your health.

Suggested Menus

The following menus are for use both during and after the detoxification period. Note that the cup you should use for the measures given below is an eight-ounce measure, not a full mug.

Day 1

Breakfast:	Oatmeal made with water, raw honey and soy milk
Snack:	⅓ cup pecans
Lunch:	Vegetable Paella (page 250)
Snack:	2 kiwi fruit
Dinner:	Rice Pilaf (page 251) and Fig Bars (page 270)
Snack:	Banana

Day 2

Breakfast:	Grapefruit and 2 slices whole-grain toast
Snack:	⅛ cup sunflower seeds
Lunch:	Artichoke Salad (page 260) and 2 rye crispbreads
Snack:	Raw carrots and celery with fat-free dip
Dinner:	Grilled wild salmon with lemon, potatoes, broccoli and peas
Snack:	⅓ cup cashews

Day 3

Breakfast:	Wedge of cantaloupe
Snack:	⅓ cup mixed dried fruit and nuts
Lunch:	Tomato and Orange Soup (page 220), whole-grain roll, and 2 Farmhouse Cookies (page 265)
Snack:	Dried apricots
Dinner:	Homemade vegetable curry and brown rice
Snack:	Apple

Day 4

Breakfast:	Bircher Muesli (page 219) with rice milk
Snack:	Orange
Lunch:	Falafel, pear
Snack:	2 rye crispbreads with cottage cheese
Dinner:	Chicken Rolls (page 252) with potatoes, green beans and carrots
Snack:	Raw carrots, celery and virtually fat-free dip

Day 5

Breakfast:	Fresh fruit salad
Snack:	⅓ cup pecans
Lunch:	Modern Ratatouille (page 251) with millet and Lemon Mousse (page 261)
Snack:	2 oatcakes
Dinner:	2 soft-boiled eggs on whole-grain toast and Banana Split (page 263)
Snack:	Slice of Carrot Cake (page 269)

Day 6

Breakfast:	Oatmeal with cracked flaxseed, molasses and soy milk
Snack:	½ cup dried fruit
Lunch:	Baked sweet potato with cottage cheese and pineapple and 2 Oatie Bran Fingers (page 271)
Snack:	Banana
Dinner:	Pasta 'n' Fish (page 254) and an apple
Snack:	⅓ cup cashews

Day 7

Breakfast:	Whole-grain toast with raw honey
Snack:	Orange
Lunch:	Avocado and Cheese (page 253) with salad and fresh fruit salad
Snack:	¼ cup toasted sesame seeds with Kelpamare seasoning
Dinner:	Cajun Fish Filets (page 243) and No-fry Fries (page 242)
Snack:	1–2 slice(s) whole-grain bread with peanut butter

Besides being organically grown, the foods used in these menus should be additive and preservative-free. Do not forget to bring in the other foods recommended, however, so that, all in all, you consume a wide variety of foods. The recipes that follow should add further variety.

PART III

Healing Recipes

As already discussed, healthy eating is fundamental to relieving the myriad symptoms of fibromyalgia. It is also the first line of defense against further invasive disease. This part of the book is devoted to recipes using foods that are known to aid the healing process.

ESSENTIAL BASICS

Homemade Vegetable Stock

Makes 1 pint

- 1 tbsp sunflower oil
- 1 potato, chopped
- 1 carrot, chopped
- 1 onion, chopped
- 1 celery stick, chopped
- 2 garlic cloves, peeled
- 4 parsley stalks
- 1 sprig thyme
- 1 bay leaf
- pinch of freshly ground black pepper
- 1 pint filtered water

Heat the sunflower oil in a large saucepan, then add the vegetables. Cover and boil gently for about 10 minutes. Add the herbs, mix and pour the water into the pan. Bring back to a boil, then simmer, partially covered, for 40 minutes. Strain, season with the pepper and use as required. This stock will add flavor to stews and soups or may simply be poured over your steamed vegetables. It can be frozen or stored in a refrigerator for 3–4 days.

Basic Meat Sauce

Serves 8

Submitted by Dorothy Holden

1½ lbs lean minced beef or lamb

4 oz lean back bacon

2 onions, finely chopped

1 garlic clove, crushed

4 oz carrots, finely diced

1 green bell pepper, deseeded and finely diced

4 oz mushrooms, sliced

2 celery sticks, chopped

14-oz can chopped tomatoes, including juice

3 oz tomato purée

pinch of sea salt or to taste

pinch of freshly ground black pepper

1 oz basil, chopped

½ tbsp vegetable stock or Homemade Vegetable Stock (page 214)

½ tbsp corn flour

Place the mince in a large saucepan and sauté (that is, cover and allow to cook in its own steam) over a low heat until it starts to turn brown. Add the bacon, onions, garlic, carrots, pepper, mushrooms and celery, stirring all the time. Add the canned tomatoes, juice and all, and the tomato purée, then season with salt, pepper and basil. Cover and simmer gently for half an hour. Gradually add the stock and flour, stirring well until the desired consistency is achieved. This meat sauce can be frozen when it has cooled.

Savory Curry Sauce

Serves 4

Cooked red meat, poultry or frozen seafood can be added to this sauce.

Submitted by Dorothy Holden

> 2 large onions, finely chopped
>
> 4 garlic cloves or to taste, crushed
>
> 1 tsp coriander, fresh or dried
>
> ½ pint filtered water, approximately
>
> 2 tsp ground cumin
>
> 1 tbsp olive oil
>
> 1 tsp chili powder
>
> 2 tsp turmeric
>
> 1 tsp garam masala
>
> 4 tsp paprika
>
> 2 tsp dried fenugreek leaves
>
> 1 tbsp tomato purée
>
> 1 tbsp tomato ketchup
>
> pinch of sea salt or to taste

Place the onions and garlic in a frying pan and sauté over a medium heat for 5 minutes. Keeping back a little coriander, mix the spices into a jug of ¼ pint of the water, then add to the pan. Cook for another 5 minutes, then reduce the heat to a simmer. Add the tomato purée, the ketchup and a little more water, then simmer for about 20 minutes. Keep adding water so it does not become too dry. Add the precooked meat, chicken or frozen seafood, if using, together with a pinch of salt, and heat through, stirring all the time. Serve garnished with the remaining coriander. Remember that meat should only be eaten two to three times a week.

Whole-grain Shortcrust Pastry

Makes 1 pound

> 4 oz plain organic whole-grain flour
> 4 oz self-raising organic whole-grain flour
> 4 oz butter
> a pinch of sea salt or to taste
> 4 fl oz filtered water

Place the flours, butter and salt in a bowl. Rub the butter into the flour until the mixture resembles fine breadcrumbs. Gradually add the water and mix with a round-ended knife to form a soft dough, then draw together with the fingertips. Leave the dough in the bowl and refrigerate for 5 minutes. Then, roll it out on a floured surface and use as required. Because of its high butter content, try to make this pastry a treat!

Oatmeal Pastry

Makes 1 pound

> 6 oz self-rising organic flour
> 2 oz fine oat flour
> 5 oz butter
> 2 oz light brown sugar

Place the flours and butter in a bowl. Rub the butter in with the fingertips to keep the fat cool. Add the sugar and mix it in with the hands. A little water may be required to bind the mixture to form a dough. Roll it out on a floured surface and use as required. Again, this pastry should be eaten sparingly.

BREAKFASTS

Breakfast Banana

Serves 2–3

> 3 small bananas
> 2 tsp fresh lemon juice
> pinch ground cinnamon
> 2 oz uncoated cashew nuts, finely chopped or ground

Mash 1 banana in a bowl, adding the lemon juice. If required, add a little filtered water to make a smooth paste. Add the cinnamon. Now slice the other bananas and mix into the sauce. Spoon into dessert glasses and garnish with the nuts.

Sweet Potato Beginnings

Serves 3–4

> 2 sweet potatoes, pierced
> 2 bananas, sliced
> 1 apple, peeled, cored and diced
> ½ tsp ground cinnamon

Bake the sweet potatoes in the microwave on high for 5 to 7 minutes or until soft. Allow to stand until cool enough to touch, then peel and mash in a bowl. Add the fruit and stir well. Sprinkle with cinnamon and serve hot.

Bircher Muesli

Serves 2

1 apple, coarsely chopped

3 oz raisins, washed

1 orange, segmented and chopped

1 banana, chopped

5 oz rolled oats

3–5 fl oz soy or rice milk, to taste

Place all the ingredients in a medium bowl and mix together. Serve.

SOUPS

Tomato and Orange Soup

Serves 6

    8 oz potatoes, diced

    1 large onion, finely chopped

    1 lb tomatoes, blanched, peeled and quartered

    1 pint vegetable stock or Homemade Vegetable Stock (page 214)

    peel and juice of 1 orange

    ½ tsp dried oregano, chopped

    pinch of sea salt or to taste

    pinch of freshly ground black pepper or to taste

    1 orange, quartered

    3 slices toasted whole-grain bread, diced to make croutons

Place the potatoes, onion, tomatoes, stock, orange peel and juice, oregano, salt and pepper in a large saucepan. Bring to a boil, cover and simmer gently for 30 minutes. Place in a blender or food processor and blend well, sieving to remove any seeds. Return to the pan and reheat, adding a little more stock if required. Ladle into warmed bowls, garnishing each with a segment of orange and sprinkle the croutons over.

Gazpacho (Chilled Soup)

Serves 4

1 lb tomatoes, roughly sliced

1 onion, diced

1 green bell pepper, deseeded and diced

1 garlic clove, crushed

1 tbsp olive oil

1 tbsp organic apple cider vinegar

juice of 1 lemon

¼ cucumber, diced

pinch of sea salt or to taste

pinch of freshly ground black pepper or to taste

3 slices toasted whole-grain bread, diced to make croutons

Place the tomatoes, onion, pepper, garlic, olive oil and vinegar in a blender and combine well. Pour the mixture into a bowl, adding the lemon juice and salt and pepper to taste. Chill in a refrigerator before serving with croutons.

Carrot Borscht

Serves 4

1 onion, finely chopped

1 large potato, peeled and diced

1 tsp olive oil

1 raw beetroot, peeled and diced

12 oz carrots, peeled and diced

3 cups Homemade Vegetable Stock (page 214)

8 oz soft tofu, squeezed to remove excess liquid (optional)

¼ tsp ground nutmeg

pinch of sea salt or to taste

pinch of freshly ground black pepper or to taste

handful fresh mint, chopped

Place the onion and potato in a large saucepan and sauté very gently in the olive oil for 7 to 10 minutes, stirring frequently. Add the beetroot and carrots, cover and simmer for another 20 minutes. Pour in the stock and simmer for another 10 minutes. Add the tofu, if using, then pour the contents of the pan into a blender or food processor. After blending to a smooth consistency, adding the nutmeg and seasoning to taste, ladle the soup into warmed bowls. Garnish with the chopped mint and serve.

Tomato and Lentil Soup

Serves 4

1 large onion, finely chopped

4 tomatoes, skinned and quartered

4 oz red lentils, rinsed

9 fl oz Homemade Vegetable Stock (page 214)

pinch of sea salt or to taste

pinch of freshly ground black pepper or to taste

4 fresh basil leaves, chopped

Place the onion in a large saucepan and sauté in a little water until just softened. Add the tomatoes and lentils, then stir in the stock. Season with salt and pepper. Bring to a boil, cover and simmer gently for 30 minutes or until the lentils are tender. Remove from the heat and pour the mixture into a blender or food processor and process until smooth. Return to the pan and heat through. Ladle into warmed bowls and garnish with the basil.

Cream of Potato Soup

Serves 3

1 lb potatoes, peeled and diced

1 large onion, finely chopped

2 medium celery sticks, sliced

½ oz butter

¾ pint filtered water

pinch of sea salt or to taste

pinch of freshly ground black pepper or to taste

½ pint skimmed milk

2 tbsp chopped fresh parsley

Place the vegetables and the butter in a medium saucepan and add 1 tablespoonful of the water. Sauté very gently for 7 to 10 minutes. Add the remaining water and season. Bring to a boil, cover and simmer gently for 25 minutes. Pour the soup into a blender or food processor and mix until smooth. Return to the pan and stir in the milk. Bring to a boil once more, stirring well, then cover and simmer for 5 minutes. Ladle into warmed bowls and sprinkle with the parsley.

Cock-a-Leekie Soup

Serves 3

10 oz skinless, boned chicken, diced

2 tsp olive oil

1 tbsp filtered water

12 oz leeks, chopped into 1-inch lengths, green parts finely
    shredded

2 pints vegetable stock or Homemade Vegetable Stock (page 214)

1 bouquet of fresh herbs, such as thyme, sage and rosemary

6 prunes, pitted and halved

3 sprigs fresh parsley

Place the chicken, olive oil and water in a medium saucepan and gently sauté until the chicken has browned a little on all sides. Add the white pieces of leek to the pan and continue to cook for another 5 minutes, until the leeks have softened. Add the stock and herb bouquet. Bring to a boil, then simmer for 30 minutes. Add the green leek pieces and prunes. Simmer for 30 more minutes. Ladle into warmed bowls and garnish with the parsley.

Cabbage and Leek Soup

Serves 6

>   2 pints vegetable stock or Homemade Vegetable Stock (page 214)
>   8 leeks, trimmed, washed and diced
>   2¾ lbs green or Savoy cabbage, stalk and outer leaves removed, rest chopped into ¾-inch pieces
>   1 large onion, finely chopped
>   pinch of sea salt or to taste
>   pinch of freshly ground black pepper or to taste
>   6 slices Granary bread, toasted and diced to make croutons
>   2 oz low-fat organic Cheddar cheese, grated (optional)

Pour the stock into a large saucepan and bring to a boil. Add the vegetables, then bring back to a boil. Cover and simmer gently for 35–45 minutes, stirring occasionally. Season with the salt and pepper. Ladle into warmed bowls, garnish with the croutons and sprinkle the cheese over the top, if using.

MAIN MEALS

Microwave Chili Con Carne

Serves 4

Submitted by Dorothy Holden

Basic Meat Sauce (page 215)

1 green bell pepper, deseeded and thinly sliced

1 tbsp olive oil

1 tbsp red wine vinegar

1 tsp light or dark brown sugar

1–2 tsp chili powder, according to taste

1 tbsp ground cumin

1 medium can red kidney beans, drained

Reheat the meat sauce from frozen in a microwave by setting it for 10 minutes on "defrost," then cook on high for 1½ minutes. Allow to stand. Place the pepper in a frying pan and sauté in the olive oil for about 3 minutes or until softened. Stir in the vinegar, sugar, chili powder and cumin. Mix well. Add to the meat sauce. Add the kidney beans. Cover and microwave on a medium setting for 5 minutes or until heated through.

Microwave Chicken Curry

Serves 4

Submitted by Dorothy Holden

> 1 lb brown rice
>
> 1 onion, finely chopped
>
> 1 tbsp sunflower oil
>
> 1–2 tbsp medium madras curry powder or to taste
>
> 1 tbsp corn flour
>
> 1 pint vegetable stock or Homemade Vegetable Stock (page 214)
>
> 1 tsp Worcestershire sauce
>
> 2 tsp tomato purée
>
> 2 tsp fresh lemon juice
>
> 2 tsp mango chutney
>
> 1 dessert apple, peeled, cored and sliced
>
> 2 oz golden raisins, washed
>
> 12 oz cooked chicken, diced
>
> pinch of sea salt or to taste
>
> pinch of freshly ground black pepper or to taste

Bring a large pan of water to a boil, stir in the rice, cover, reduce the heat and simmer for 30 minutes until tender. Toward the end of the cooking time for the rice, place the onion and sunflower oil in a microwavable dish. Cover and microwave on high for 1½ minutes, then stir. Add the curry powder and corn flour and, stirring well, gradually blend in the stock. Re-cover and microwave on high for 3 minutes or until the sauce has boiled and thickened. Stir, add the Worcestershire sauce, tomato purée, lemon juice, chutney, apple and raisins and stir again. Cover and microwave on high for 2 minutes. Add the chicken, salt and pepper, then stir and re-cover. Microwave on high for a final 2 minutes or until piping hot. Serve on a ring of the brown rice. When cooled, this sauce can be frozen for later use.

Bavarian Beef Stew

Serves 5

> 1 lb lean beef, or lamb, stewing meat, diced into 1-inch pieces
>
> 1 tbsp sunflower or other light oil
>
> 1 large onion, finely chopped
>
> ¾ tsp caraway seeds
>
> pinch of sea salt or to taste
>
> pinch of freshly ground black pepper or to taste
>
> 1 bay leaf
>
> 7 fl oz cider vinegar
>
> ¼ tbsp fructose
>
> ½ small head red cabbage, cut into 4 wedges
>
> 7 fl oz vegetable stock or Homemade Vegetable Stock (page 214)
>
> 2 oz crushed gingersnap cookies

Place the meat and oil in a heavy-bottomed frying pan and sauté until just turning brown. Remove the meat and sauté the onion in the remaining oil until golden. Return the meat to the pan and add the stock, caraway seeds, salt, pepper and bay leaf. Bring to a boil then cover and simmer gently for 1¼ hours. Add the cider vinegar and fructose, stirring well. Place the cabbage on top of the meat. Cover and simmer for 20 minutes or until the cabbage is tender. Arrange the meat and cabbage on a platter and keep warm. Pour the stock into a small saucepan and add the crushed ginger snaps. Stirring well, cook until thickened. Serve with the meat and vegetables.

Autumn Mashed Potatoes

Serves 6

    8 oz carrots, thinly sliced
    1½ lbs potatoes, peeled and diced
    1 small rutabaga, peeled and diced
    3 parsnips, peeled and diced
    2 fl oz skimmed milk
    1 oz butter
    pinch of sea salt or to taste
    pinch of freshly ground black pepper or to taste
    1 oz chopped chives
    2 sprigs fresh mint (optional)

Place the carrots in a saucepan of boiling water and simmer for 5 minutes.
Add the potatoes, rutabaga and parsnips, cover, then simmer for 10 to
15 more minutes or until the vegetables are tender. Drain and mash
together, adding the milk, butter, salt and pepper. Spoon into a serving
bowl and sprinkle the chives over. Garnish with the mint and serve.

Sweet and Sour Chicken with Brown Rice

Serves 2–3

Submitted by David Craggs-Hinton

3 oz brown rice, cooked

6 oz chicken breast, skinned and cut into thin strips

pinch of sea salt or to taste

pinch of freshly ground black pepper or to taste

1 tsp olive oil

½ oz ginger root, peeled and grated

2–3 sprigs fresh coriander

¼ tsp Chinese five spice powder

1 garlic clove, crushed

2 tsp light brown sugar

½ pint filtered water

2 oz green beans, sliced

2 oz carrots, cut into 2-inch-long sticks

2 oz white cabbage, cut into 2-inch-long strips

2 oz bean sprouts, cut diagonally into 1-inch lengths

1 oz water chestnuts, sliced

2 tsp cider vinegar

1 tbsp soy sauce

½ oz fresh basil, chopped, or pinch dried

Place the chicken strips in a wok or frying pan and season with salt and pepper. Add the olive oil, cover and sauté for 5 minutes. Add the ginger, coriander, Chinese five spice powder, garlic, sugar and half of the water. Bring to a boil and simmer gently for 5 minutes. Remove the chicken and keep warm. Now add to the pan the green beans, carrots, cabbage, bean sprouts, water chestnuts, cider vinegar and soy sauce to taste. Gradually pour in the remaining water, stirring well. Cover and cook until the vegetables are soft and the stock has reduced. Add the chicken once more and stir well. Serve on a ring of brown rice and garnish with the chopped basil.

Salmon with Spinach and Pasta

Serves 2–3

Submitted by David Craggs-Hinton

> 2 x 4-oz salmon steaks
>
> 2 pinches sea salt or to taste
>
> pinch of freshly ground black pepper or to taste
>
> ½ oz butter
>
> 18 fl oz skim milk or rice milk
>
> 2 sprigs fresh basil or pinch dried mixed herbs
>
> 6 oz fresh spinach, finely chopped
>
> 2 tsp corn flour
>
> 6 oz whole-grain pasta, cooked, drained and rinsed
>
> 1 oz Parmesan cheese or to taste, finely grated
>
> 2 sprigs fresh parsley

Place the salmon in a medium saucepan, add a pinch of salt, pepper, the butter, half of the milk and the basil or mixed herbs, cover and poach for 15 to 20 minutes or until the salmon is cooked. Place the spinach in a medium saucepan with a pinch of salt, cover with water, bring to a boil, cover and simmer for 10 minutes. Remove the salmon from the milk and keep warm. Pour the remaining milk into the pan, add the corn flour and bring to a boil, stirring continuously, until the sauce thickens. Drain the spinach and add to the hot pasta. Add the sauce to the pasta and spinach and stir well. Garnish each serving with a sprinkling of Parmesan cheese and a sprig of parsley. Serve.

Tunisian Vegetable Couscous

Serves 6–8

- 10 oz whole wheat couscous
- 14 fl oz boiling filtered water
- 1 large onion, finely chopped
- 2 garlic cloves, crushed
- 2 tbsp white wine
- 16-oz can tomatoes, chopped
- 3 large carrots, cut into 1-inch long sticks
- 2 large celery sticks, cut into 1-inch long sticks
- 1 medium turnip, cut into ½-inch dice
- ½ tsp ground cinnamon
- ½ tsp turmeric
- 1 tsp paprika
- pinch cayenne pepper or to taste
- 2 tsp dark corn syrup
- ½ lb eggplant, cut into 1-inch strips
- 1 red bell pepper, deseeded and chopped
- 3 oz raisins
- 5 oz dried apricots, chopped
- 11-oz can chickpeas, drained and rinsed
- 4 sprigs fresh mint or parsley, chopped

Place the couscous in a large bowl and add the boiling water. Let it stand for 15 minutes, then fluff with a fork and keep warm. Sauté the onion and garlic in the wine until limp. Add the tomatoes and their liquid, carrots, celery, turnip, spices and corn syrup and bring to a boil. Cover and simmer for about 20 minutes. Add the eggplant, red pepper, raisins, apricots and chickpeas. Cover and simmer for an additional 15 minutes. Place the couscous in individual soup bowls and top with the vegetable stew. Garnish with the chopped mint or parsley.

Pesto Sauce for Pasta

Serves 4–6

> 8 oz whole-grain pasta, cooked and drained
>
> 2 large garlic cloves, raw or roasted
>
> 2 tbsp olive oil
>
> 1 large bunch fresh basil leaves
>
> 3 oz shelled walnuts
>
> 1 tbsp soy sauce
>
> 8–14 tbsp filtered water, as required
>
> pinch of sea salt or to taste
>
> pinch of freshly ground black pepper or to taste

Place the garlic and olive oil in a blender or food processor and mix until the garlic has been pulverized. Add the remaining ingredients to the blender or food processor, keeping back a few sprigs of basil. Using 8 tablespoons of water, blend the mixture until smooth, adding more water as required. Pour over the hot whole-grain pasta, garnishing with the remaining basil. Serve.

Spaghetti Balls

Serves 4–6

20 oz whole-grain spaghetti

12 oz tofu, squeezed to remove liquid

1 small onion, finely chopped

2 oz whole-grain breadcrumbs

1½ tbsp unsweetened peanut butter

2 tbsp soy sauce

1 garlic clove, crushed

½ tsp mustard powder

1 tbsp filtered water

pinch of freshly ground black pepper or to taste

2 tsp olive oil

½ oz fresh parsley, finely chopped

Bring a large pan of water to a boil, add the spaghetti, stirring, once the strands have softened, to separate them. Cook for about 10 to 15 minutes until tender, then drain. Meanwhile, place the tofu in a mixing bowl and mash with a fork. Using a wooden spoon, mix in all the other ingredients, except for the oil and a little of the parsley. Coat a heavy-bottomed frying pan with the olive oil and heat. Shape the mixture into small balls and brown on all sides over a medium heat. Drain on a paper towel and serve on the pasta. Garnish with the remaining parsley.

Fettuccine with Lentil Sauce

Serves 4

> 1 lb dried or fresh fettuccine or tagliatelle
>
> 2 tbsp olive oil
>
> 2 garlic cloves, crushed
>
> 1 large onion, finely chopped
>
> 8 oz red lentils, washed and drained
>
> 3 tbsp tomato purée
>
> ½ pint boiling filtered water
>
> pinch of sea salt or to taste
>
> pinch of freshly ground black pepper or to taste
>
> 4 sprigs fresh parsley, chopped

Place the pasta in a large saucepan, cover with water and cook according to the directions on the packaging. Drain, rinse and set aside. Heat the olive oil, then sauté the garlic and onion for 2 minutes, stirring occasionally. Add the lentils, tomato purée, salt and pepper, then stir in the boiling water. Bring to a boil, cover and simmer, stirring occasionally, for about 20 minutes or until the lentils are soft. Add more water if it looks too dry. Season with the salt and pepper. Reheat the pasta if necessary, then serve topped with the sauce. Garnish with the parsley.

Baked Macaroni with Bechamel Sauce

Serves 4

- 1 lb whole-grain macaroni, cooked
- 3 tbsp sunflower or sesame oil
- 2 medium onions, chopped
- 1 large carrot, sliced into 1-inch-long sticks
- 3 tbsp organic whole-grain flour
- ¾ pint filtered water
- ½ lb firm tofu, drained and crumbled
- 4 tbsp soy sauce or to taste
- 1 tbsp toasted sesame seeds (optional)
- 4 sprigs fresh thyme, chopped

Preheat the oven to 350°F. Heat the oil in a large saucepan and sauté the onions and carrot for 5 minutes, until the onions have become transparent and lightly browned. Lower the heat and gradually stir in the flour. Brown lightly for 30 seconds, stirring constantly. Slowly pour in the water, stirring all the time to prevent lumps forming. Return to a medium heat and cook, stirring until smooth and thickened. Now stir in the tofu and season with soy sauce. Place the cooked macaroni in a large casserole dish and stir in the vegetables and sauce, making sure the macaroni is all coated with sauce. Top with sesame seeds, if using. Cover and cook in the preheated oven for 20 minutes. Remove the lid and cook for another 20 minutes. Take out of the oven and allow to rest for 10 minutes before serving. Garnish with the chopped thyme.

Almond and Mushroom Casserole

Serves 4

- ½ lb whole-grain pasta, cooked
- 5 tbsp sunflower oil
- 2 tbsp organic whole-grain flour
- 8 fl oz unsweetened soy milk
- 2 tbsp chopped fresh parsley
- 1 tsp fresh lemon juice
- ½ tsp celery salt
- ½ lb firm tofu, squeezed to remove excess water
- ½ lb mushrooms, chopped
- ½ large green bell pepper, deseeded and finely chopped
- ½ lb blanched flaked almonds
- 4 oz whole-grain breadcrumbs

Preheat the oven to 375°F. Heat 3 tablespoons of the oil in a large saucepan over a medium heat. Add the flour, stirring until it absorbs the oil and is just starting to brown. Gradually pour in the milk, stirring or whisking constantly to avoid lumps forming. Continue cooking and stirring until the sauce begins to thicken. Remove from the heat and stir in the parsley, lemon juice and celery salt. Crumble in the tofu, mixing well, then set the sauce aside. Heat the remaining oil in a small frying pan, adding the mushrooms and sautéing until tender. Mix the mushrooms, green pepper, almonds and cooked pasta into the sauce. Transfer the mixture to a casserole dish, spreading evenly. Sprinkle the breadcrumbs over the pasta mixture and bake in the preheated oven for about 20 minutes. Remove when the top has lightly browned. Serve hot.

Pasta Oregano

Serves 2

Submitted by David Craggs-Hinton

12 oz whole-grain pasta, cooked and drained

1 small red onion, finely chopped

2 tsp olive oil

1½ lbs fresh plum tomatoes, roughly chopped

1 red bell pepper, deseeded and chopped

1 orange bell pepper, deseeded and chopped

2 oz green olives, pitted and chopped

1–2 garlic cloves to taste

½ tsp dried oregano

2 tsp tomato purée

½ tbsp organic cider vinegar

pinch of sea salt or to taste

pinch of freshly ground black pepper or to taste

½ oz fresh thyme, chopped

2 oz Parmesan cheese, finely grated

Place the onion in a frying pan with the olive oil and a little of the juice from the tomatoes. Sauté until the onions have become transparent. Add the peppers, olives and garlic and cook for another 5 minutes. Add the oregano, tomatoes, tomato purée, cider vinegar, salt and pepper and bring to a boil. Simmer for 20 to 30 minutes. Top the pasta with the sauce, sprinkle with the thyme and Parmesan cheese and serve.

Pasta Primavera

Serves 4

12 oz whole-grain spaghetti, cooked and drained

2 tbsp sunflower oil

1 bunch spring onions, thinly sliced, green and white parts in
separate piles

8 oz carrots, sliced into 1-inch-long sticks

2 medium eggplants, sliced into 1-inch-long sticks

8 oz fresh or frozen garden peas

2 tbsp fresh mint leaves, chopped

pinch of sea salt or to taste

pinch of freshly ground black pepper or to taste

Heat the oil in a large saucepan over a medium heat. Add the white
parts of the spring onions and sauté very gently for 2 to 3 minutes. Add
the carrots and lower the heat. Cover and simmer for 5 minutes, then
add the eggplants and peas, covering and simmering for another 2 to 3
minutes. Turn off the heat, stir in the mint and season with salt and pepper.
Transfer the cooked vegetables to the saucepan or dish in which
you have the spaghetti and mix together. Serve hot.

Lazy Mini Pizzas

Serves 3–6

1 tbsp olive oil

1 red onion, chopped

1 tsp dried mixed herbs

1 tsp dried oregano

pinch garlic salt

3 tomatoes, peeled

6 green olives, pitted

4 oz canned kidney beans, drained and coarsely chopped

3 fresh soft whole-grain rolls, halved

pinch of sea salt or to taste

pinch of freshly ground black pepper or to taste

1½ oz Edam cheese, grated

Place the olive oil in a medium frying pan and add the onion. Sauté for 2 minutes, then add the herbs and garlic salt. Sauté for another 2 minutes, then add the tomatoes, olives and beans. Cover and simmer for 10 minutes. Toast the outsides of the rolls, then spread the tomato mixture evenly on the cut surface of each half, seasoning with the salt and pepper. Place on a baking tray, sprinkle the cheese on top of the mixture and grill until the cheese has turned golden and is bubbling. Serve, with a side salad if desired.

No-fry Fries

Serves 1–2

> 1 large potato, peeled and cut into fries

Place the "fries" on a microwave-safe plate in a radial fashion, with the end of each one pointing toward the center of the plate. Microwave on high for 2 minutes, flipping them over and removing any that are cooked. Microwave for another 2 minutes or until the chips are pliable but not too dried. Place on a lightly oiled baking tray and grill for a few minutes, turning them over so that all sides become browned. Serve hot.

Sweet Potato Fries

Serves 3

> 2 sweet potatoes (or yams), peeled and cut into fries
> olive oil as required
> ½ tsp garlic salt

Preheat the oven to 350°F. Place the fries on a lightly oiled baking tray and brush on a light coating of olive oil. Sprinkle with some of the garlic salt and bake for 20 minutes in the preheated oven. Turn the fries over, sprinkle with the remaining garlic salt and bake for another 10 minutes. Serve hot.

Cajun Fish Filets

Serves 4

> 1 lb any white fish
> 1 tsp Cajun spice
> 1 tbsp paprika
> pinch of freshly ground black pepper or to taste
> 1 lemon, quartered

Arrange the filets on a lightly oiled grill pan. Mix together the cajun spice and paprika and sprinkle over the filets so they are well coated. Grill close to the heat for 5 to 6 minutes or until the spices have browned and the fish is firm and will flake with a fork. Season with black pepper and serve with a salad, Sweet Potato Fries or No-fry Fries (page 242). Garnish with the lemon wedges.

Kedgeree

Serves 4

> 8 oz. haddock, smoked or unsmoked
> 1 small onion, finely chopped
> 1 tsp olive oil
> 6 oz organic long-grain brown rice
> pinch cayenne pepper
> 4 sprigs fresh parsley, chopped

Place the haddock in a medium saucepan and cover with water. Poach gently for 10 minutes, then drain, reserving the liquid. Remove the bones and skin from the fish, flaking the flesh loosely with a fork. Sauté the onion in the oil until soft, add the rice and cayenne pepper, then stir for a few more seconds. Mix in the liquid from the fish and simmer until the rice is tender (about 30 minutes) adding more water if required. Stir frequently. Gently add the flaked haddock and mix together. Turn on to a heated dish, garnish with the parsley and serve.

Caribbean Pork and Pineapple

Serves 2–3

    6 oz brown rice, cooked
    10 oz pork tenderloin, chopped into large dice
    4 oz onion, finely chopped
    4 oz mushrooms, sliced
    4 oz pineapple cubes in natural juice
    ¼ pint vegetable stock or Homemade Vegetable Stock (page 214)
    ¼ pint tomato juice
    ½ oz fresh ginger root, peeled and finely chopped (optional)
    2 sprigs fresh basil

Place the pork and onions in a frying pan and sauté gently until the pork has sealed on all sides and the onions have softened, adding a teaspoonful of water if the onion begins to stick. Add the remaining ingredients, except the basil, cover and simmer for 20 to 5 minutes. Serve on a ring of brown rice and garnish with the basil.

Beef Casserole

Serves 4

    1 lb lean braising steak, cut into strips
    12 oz carrots, sliced
    8 oz leeks, sliced
    12 oz rutabaga
    4 oz pearl barley
    1½ pints vegetable stock or Homemade Vegetable Stock (page 214)
    pinch of sea salt or to taste

Preheat the oven to 325°F, Place all the ingredients in a saucepan, cover with water and bring to a boil. Skim the excess fat from the top, then stir and place in a casserole dish. Cover and cook in the preheated oven for 1½ to 2 hours. Serve with the baked potato and green beans.

Chicken Burgers

Serves 4

> 8 oz cooked chicken breast, minced
> 1 small onion, grated
> small pinch of sea salt
> pinch of freshly ground black pepper or to taste
> 10 oz cottage cheese, sieved to remove the liquid
> 1 tsp mixed herbs

Place the chicken and the onion in a medium mixing bowl and mix together. Season with salt and pepper. Stir in the cottage cheese and mixed herbs, then make into 4 burger shapes. Leave to cool in a refrigerator for 1 to 2 hours before cooking under a hot grill for about 5 minutes each side or until the burgers are a golden color. Serve with a salad.

Eggplant with Chicken Strips

Serves 4

> 1 tsp coriander seeds, roasted and finely ground
>
> 1 tsp fennel seeds, roasted and finely ground
>
> 1 garlic clove, crushed
>
> 1 tsp grated fresh ginger root
>
> pinch of sea salt or to taste
>
> pinch of freshly ground black pepper or to taste
>
> 2 tbsp olive oil, plus extra for eggplant
>
> 12 oz chicken filet, cut into thin strips
>
> 3, 5-inch-long eggplants, sliced in half and cut into strips length-
>   wise
>
> ½ tsp tamari
>
> 2 tsp brown rice vinegar

Preheat the oven to 400°F. Combine the coriander and fennel seeds, garlic, ginger, salt and pepper with the olive oil in a blender or food processor. Mix until smooth. Half fill a large saucepan with water and bring to a boil. Blanch the chicken strips for 20 seconds, then immediately drain in a colander and plunge into a large bowl of ice-cold water. Leave in the cold water for about 10 minutes or until the strips have completely cooled. Drain again. Stir the chicken into the spicy oil mixture, then place in the refrigerator to marinate for at least 30 minutes. Slice each piece of eggplant across diagonally and rub with a little olive oil. Arrange them in a single layer in a large, lightly oiled ovenproof dish. Fill the gaps with the marinated chicken strips. Cook in the preheated oven for 7 to 8 minutes. Turn the oven off without opening the door and leave the dish to stand for another 3 to 4 minutes. Ensure the chicken strips are cooked through. Sprinkle with the tamari and rice vinegar, then serve while still hot with a salad or steamed vegetables.

Spinach and Lentil Stew

Serves 5

1 onion, chopped

2 fl oz Homemade Vegetable Stock (page 214)

4 garlic cloves, finely chopped

6 oz split red lentils, rinsed

14-oz can chopped tomatoes, with juice

4 tsp boullion granules

1 tbsp Worcestershire sauce

1 tsp dried thyme

½ tsp ground fennel seeds (optional)

1 bay leaf

pinch of sea salt or to taste

2 medium carrots, diced

10 oz fresh spinach, chopped

1½ pints filtered water

1 tbsp organic apple cider vinegar

Place the onion in a large saucepan and sauté in the vegetable stock until soft (3 to 4 minutes). Add the garlic, lentils, tomatoes and juice, stock granules, Worcestershire sauce, thyme, fennel seeds, if using, bay leaf and salt, together with the water. Bring to a boil, cover and, stirring occasionally, simmer for 20 minutes or until the lentils start to break up. Add the carrots and spinach and stir well (if the spinach was frozen, stir until it has thawed). Cover and simmer for another 15 minutes or until the carrots and spinach are cooked. Remove the bay leaf and stir in the vinegar. Serve hot.

Potato Gnocchi

Serves 4

> 3 large baking potatoes,
> 5 oz organic whole-grain, self-raising flour
> ½ tsp sea salt

Bake or microwave the potatoes until tender, allowing them to rest at room temperature until they are cool enough to handle. Scoop the potato out of the skins and mash in a bowl. Add the flour and salt, mixing in well, then turn the mixture on to a floured surface. Knead until smooth, adding more flour if necessary so the "dough" does not stick. Bring a large saucepan of water to a boil. Form the dough into ¾-inch-thick sausages, then cut across at ¾-inch intervals. Press the top of each shape lightly with a fork to create stripes. Add the gnocchi to the boiling water, boiling until they float to the top. Remove them from the water and drain well. Place in a large bowl, adding sufficient Tangy Pasta Sauce (page 249) to lightly coat all the gnocchi. Serve with additional Tangy Pasta Sauce.

Tangy Pasta Sauce

Serves 4

> 1 tbsp olive oil
> 1 onion, finely chopped
> 1 large garlic clove, crushed
> 1 bell pepper, any color, deseeded and finely chopped
> 1 small eggplant, sliced, slices cut in half
> 2¼ lbs fresh plum tomatoes, coarsely chopped
> 1 tbsp fresh basil, chopped
> pinch of sea salt or to taste
> pinch of freshly ground black pepper or to taste
> 2 tsp fresh coriander, chopped

Heat the oil in a large, heavy bottomed saucepan over a medium heat. Add the onion and garlic, then sauté for 5 minutes. Add the bell pepper and eggplant and continue to sauté until the onions have become tender. Add the tomatoes, basil, salt and pepper and simmer gently for another 25 minutes. Garnish with the chopped coriander and serve with Potato Gnocchi (page 248).

Vegetable Paella

Serves 1

2 oz brown rice

8 fl oz boiling filtered water

1 small onion, chopped

1 small green bell pepper, deseeded and chopped

2 small tomatoes, roughly chopped

1 oz mushrooms, chopped

3 tbsp sweet corn, drained if canned

½ tsp dried thyme or marjoram

1 tsp lemon juice or to taste

1 tsp soy sauce or to taste

pinch of freshly ground black pepper or to taste

1 oz peanuts, crushed, or peanut butter (optional)

Place the rice in a medium saucepan with the boiling water. Bring back to a boil, cover and leave to simmer for 10 minutes. Add the vegetables, except the sweet corn, to the rice, stir, cover and simmer for 15 minutes. Stir in the sweet corn, herbs, lemon juice and soy sauce. Season with the pepper, cover and simmer for another 5 minutes. If using peanut butter, stir it in at this point. If using peanuts, sprinkle them on top of the dish. Serve hot.

Modern Ratatouille

Serves 4–6

1 onion, chopped

1 green bell pepper, deseeded and chopped

4 garlic cloves, crushed

6 large tomatoes, peeled and deseeded

2 tsp allspice

3 fl oz Homemade Vegetable Stock (page 214), plus extra as
     required

4 medium eggplants, sliced

½ oz fresh basil, chopped, or pinch dried

juice of 1 lemon

Place the onion, pepper and garlic in a wok or large frying pan and
sauté for 5 minutes or until soft. Add the tomatoes, allspice and stock.
Cover and simmer for 20 minutes, stirring occasionally and adding
more stock if necessary. Add the eggplants, basil and lemon juice and
simmer for another 5–10 minutes, until the eggplant has become tender
but is still bright. Serve.

Rice Pilaf

Serves 2

6 fl oz vegetable or chicken broth

6 oz long-grain brown rice

1 oz diced celery

1 oz deseeded and diced green bell pepper

1 small onion, finely chopped

2 tbsp fresh parsley, chopped

Place the stock, rice, celery, pepper and onion in a large saucepan and
bring to a boil. Cover and simmer for 20 minutes or until all the liquid
has been absorbed and the rice is tender. Stir in the parsley just before
serving.

Chicken Rolls

Serves 2

Submitted by Margaret Gray

    1 slice whole-grain bread

    1 tbsp filtered water

    1 small onion, finely chopped

    1 tsp fresh sage or pinch dried

    pinch of sea salt or to taste

    pinch of freshly ground black pepper or to taste

    1 small organic free-range egg

    2 chicken filets, skinned, washed and patted dry

Preheat the oven to 475°F. Place the bread in a bowl and rub until small crumbs are formed. Add the water and set aside. Microwave the onion on high for 2 minutes or until it has softened, then drain. Make a hollow in the bread crumb mixture and add the onion, sage, salt and pepper and mix well. Add the egg and mix again. Place the chicken pieces in a lightly oiled ovenproof dish and spread the bread mixture generously on top. Roll the chicken, making sure that the "stuffing" stays in the middle, and secure with cocktail sticks or string. Bake in the preheated oven for about 15 minutes or until the chicken is tender. Serve with steamed vegetables.

Avocado and Cheese

Serves 2–4

Submitted by Margaret Gray

  2 ripe avocados
  4 oz cottage cheese
  1 tbsp fat-free mayonnaise
  7-oz can salmon or tuna
  ½ small onion, finely chopped
  ½ tsp freshly squeezed lemon juice
  pinch paprika
  1 hard-boiled free-range egg, sliced
  mixed green salad and whole-grain rolls to serve

Cut the avocados in half lengthwise, remove the stone and spoon out the flesh into a bowl, leaving just the skins—set these to one side. Add the cottage cheese, mayonnaise, fish, onion and lemon juice to the bowl with the avocado and mix together with either a fork or blender until smooth. Spoon the mixture into the skins. Sprinkle with the paprika and garnish with the egg slices. Serve with a mixed green salad and whole-grain rolls.

Avocado Vinaigrette

Serves 4

  4 tsp organic apple cider vinegar
  6 tbsp olive oil
  pinch of sea salt or to taste
  pinch of freshly ground black pepper or to taste
  2 ripe avocados

Place the vinegar, olive oil and seasonings in a bowl and mix together. Chill in the refrigerator until ready to serve. Cut the avocados in half lengthwise and remove the stones. Place on plates and fill the hollows with the vinaigrette. Serve as a starter or with a salad.

Pasta 'n' Fish

Serves 2

Submitted by Margaret Gray

    8 oz fresh haddock or cod

    soy or rice milk as required

    4 oz whole-grain pasta

    4 oz low-fat organic cheese, grated

Preheat the oven to 450°F. Poach the fish in a little soy or rice milk, enough to cover. Remove any skin and bones, flake and set to one side. Add the pasta to a pan of boiling water and simmer for 12 minutes. Place the fish and pasta in an ovenproof dish and mix together. Stir in the cheese, saving some for later. Place in the preheated oven and bake for 5–10 minutes or until the cheese has melted and the top browned. Sprinkle the remaining cheese over the top and serve with the Homemade Coleslaw (page 255) and salad.

Homemade Coleslaw

Serves 4 to 8

Submitted by Margaret Gray

> ½ small white cabbage, finely chopped
>
> 1 small carrot, finely chopped
>
> 1 celery stick, finely chopped
>
> 1 oz raisins or nuts
>
> 6–8 oz fat-free mayonnaise

Place the dry ingredients in a bowl and mix well. Add the mayonnaise and stir again.

Stuffed Eggs

Serves 2–4

Submitted by Margaret Gray

> 4 eggs, soft-boiled and shelled
>
> 7-oz can sardines or tuna
>
> 1 tbsp fat-free mayonnaise
>
> pinch of sea salt or to taste
>
> pinch of freshly ground black pepper or to taste
>
> 1 oz watercress

Cut the eggs lengthwise and spoon the yolks into a bowl. Add the sardines or tuna, mayonnaise, salt and pepper. Mix well, then spoon the mixture into the hollows in the egg whites, piling it up. Garnish with the watercress. Serve with a salad and whole-grain bread.

Nut Pâté

Serves 3 to 4

Submitted by Margaret Gray

2 oz almonds

2 oz sunflower seeds

2 oz cashew pieces

4–6 fl oz Homemade Vegetable Stock (page 214)

Place all the ingredients in a blender or food processor and grind to a powder. Add sufficient stock to make a paste. Place in a freezer-proof plastic container and freeze for 2 or more hours before serving. Serve with the salad, baked potatoes, bread or crackers.

Bean Pâté

Serves 3

12-oz can red kidney beans

1 garlic clove, crushed

1 tbsp tomato purée

1 tsp organic soy sauce

1 tsp fresh lemon juice

½ tsp Tabasco sauce

pinch of sea salt or to taste

pinch of freshly ground black pepper or to taste

Drain the kidney beans, reserving the liquid. Place all the beans and the rest of the ingredients in a large bowl and mash with a fork. Beat well with a wooden spoon or use a food processor. If necessary, add a little of the liquid from the beans to make the mixture into a thick paste. Adjust the seasoning to taste, then spoon into medium baking dish and chill in the refrigerator for about 30 minutes before serving. Serve with the salad or baked potato.

SALADS

Black Bean Salad

Serves 6

6 oz organic long-grain brown rice

6 fl oz vegetable stock or Homemade Vegetable Stock (page 214)

6 oz pineapple chunks, chopped

15-oz can black beans, drained and rinsed

1 red bell pepper, deseeded and diced

2 celery sticks, diced

1 medium onion, finely chopped

3 tbsp organic cider vinegar

2 tbsp olive oil

2 tsp Dijon mustard

1 tsp light or dark brown sugar or to taste

pinch of sea salt or to taste

pinch of freshly ground black pepper or to taste

Place the rice and stock in a medium saucepan and bring to a boil. Stir, cover and simmer for 30 minutes. Keep covered, but remove the pan from the heat and allow to stand for 5 minutes, then fluff with a fork. Add the pineapple, beans, pepper, celery and onion and toss to combine. Add the remaining ingredients and toss to coat the salad. Serve.

Bulgar Wheat Salad with Herbs and Walnuts

Serves 4

8 oz bulgar wheat

12 fl oz vegetable stock or Homemade Vegetable Stock (page 214)

pinch ground cumin

1 cinnamon stick

pinch cayenne pepper

pinch ground cloves

1 red bell pepper, roasted, peeled, deseeded and diced

1 yellow bell pepper, roasted, peeled, deseeded and diced

2 plum tomatoes, roasted, skinned, deseeded and diced

2 shallots, finely chopped

1 oz snow peas, topped and tailed

5 black olives, pitted and quartered

2 oz walnuts, coarsely chopped

2 tbsp chopped fresh basil, parsley and mint

2 tbsp lemon juice

2 tbsp olive oil

pinch of freshly ground black pepper or to taste

Place the bulgar wheat in a large bowl. Pour the stock into a saucepan, adding the cumin, cinnamon, cayenne pepper and ground cloves. Bring to a boil and simmer for 1 minute. Pour over the bulgar wheat and allow to stand for 30 minutes. Meanwhile, place the peppers, tomatoes, shallots, snow peas, olives, walnuts and herbs in another bowl and add the lemon juice, olive oil and black pepper. Stir well. Drain the bulgar wheat, shaking the sieve or colander well to remove excess water. Remove the cinnamon stick and pour the bulgar wheat into a large serving bowl. Stir in the fresh vegetable mixture and serve.

Tangy Sweet Potato Salad with Chickpeas

Serves 6

4 sweet potatoes, peeled and cut into 1-inch cubes

4 oz cooked or canned chickpeas, drained

1 tbsp red onion, finely chopped

1 tbsp olive oil

1 oz organic cider vinegar

1 tbsp Dijon mustard

2 tsp raw honey

2 tsp Worcestershire sauce

pinch of sea salt or to taste

pinch of freshly ground black pepper or to taste

Place the sweet potatoes in a large saucepan and cover with water. Bring to a boil, cover and simmer for 10 minutes or until just tender. Drain and set aside to cool to room temperature. Combine the cooled potatoes with the chickpeas and onion in a medium bowl. Place the remaining ingredients in a small bowl and whisk together. Spoon the dressing over the potato mixture and toss gently to coat all the ingredients.

Artichoke Salad

Serves 6

14-oz can artichoke hearts, drained and sliced
3 large tomatoes, sliced
1 green bell pepper, deseeded and diced
½ oz fresh parsley, finely chopped, or pinch dried
6 tbsp olive oil
2 tbsp organic cider vinegar
1 garlic clove, crushed
pinch of sea salt or to taste
pinch of freshly ground black pepper or to taste

Place the artichoke hearts in a salad bowl with the tomatoes and pepper. Season to taste. Mix the remaining ingredients together in another small bowl. Pour over the salad and chill for 10 minutes before serving.

DESSERTS

Lemon Mousse

Serves 8

> 18 fl oz pineapple juice
>
> 3 fl oz orange juice concentrate
>
> 3 oz arrowroot
>
> 1 tbsp lemon peel
>
> 6 tbsp lemon juice
>
> 6 tbsp honey or to taste
>
> 1 tbsp orange peel, cut into thin strips
>
> ¼ tsp sea salt

Combine all the ingredients in a blender or food processor and mix until smooth. Pour the mixture into a saucepan and bring to a boil. Cover and simmer for 6 to 7 minutes, until thick, stirring all the time. Place in dessert glasses and chill in the refrigerator until cold and set. Serve.

Fruity Rice Pudding

Serves 3–4

> 6 fl oz rice milk
> 6 oz brown rice, cooked
> 3 oz raisins
> 3 oz dried apricots, chopped
> ¼ tsp ground cinnamon
> pinch of ground cloves
> pinch ground cardamom (optional)

Place the rice milk in a medium saucepan and warm over a low heat. Stir in the remaining ingredients, cover and cook, without boiling, for 15 to 20 minutes, stirring occasionally. Remove when the fruits have become plump and soft and most of the milk has been absorbed. Serve hot.

Grapefruit Cups

Serves 4

> 2 grapefruit
> 2 glacé cherries, cut in half
> ½ tsp fructose or fruit juice sweetener

Cut the grapefruit in half, then cut around each half, loosening the flesh from the outer skin. Cut between the segments to loosen the flesh, then remove the central core and pips. Place a grapefruit half in each of four individual sundae glasses. Sprinkle with a little fructose or sweetener and place half a glacé cherry in the middle of each grapefruit. Serve either as a starter or dessert.

Banana Split

Serves 2

> 2 bananas
> 4 tsp low-fat fromage frais
> 4 tsp strawberry or banana tofu yogurt
> 4 oz strawberries, hulled

Remove the skins from the bananas and cut each banana in half lengthwise. Mix together the yogurt and fromage frais and pile half in the center of each of two dessert plates. Place banana halves along each side of the mixture for both plates. Liquidize the strawberries in a blender or food processor. Pour the resulting sauce over the banana halves.

Fresh Fruit Salad

Serves 4

> 2 oz cherries, pitted
> 2 oz seedless grapes, washed
> 1 red apple, unpeeled, washed, cored and diced
> 1 green apple, unpeeled, washed, cored and diced
> 1 orange, peeled and segmented
> 2 apricots, diced
> 1 kiwi fruit, diced
> juice of 1 lemon
> 5 fl oz unsweetened apple juice

Place the cherries, grapes, apples, orange, apricots and kiwi fruit in a bowl and mix together. Pour the lemon and apple juices over the fruit and refrigerate for at least 1 hour before serving.

Baked Apple with Golden Raisins

Serves 1

> 1 medium cooking apple, washed, cored and lightly punctured
> pinch ground cinnamon
> ½ oz golden raisins

Preheat the oven to 400°F. Fill the center of the apple with raisins and sprinkle the cinnamon over. Place the apple in an ovenproof dish and pour a little water around it. Bake in the preheated oven for about 30 minutes. Allow to cool for a few minutes before serving.

CAKES AND COOKIES

Farmhouse Cookies

Makes about 20 cookies

- 6 oz organic whole-grain, self-rising flour
- 2 oz fine oatmeal
- 4 oz butter
- 1 oz light brown sugar
- 1 tsp baking powder
- ½ tsp celery salt
- ½ tsp cayenne pepper
- 1 tbsp skim milk

Preheat the oven to 350°F. Place all the dry ingredients in a bowl and mix, rubbing in the butter. Add the milk slowly, mixing until a soft dough forms. Roll out the dough on a floured surface until it is ⅛-inch thick. Using a cookie cutter, cut out shapes and place them on a lightly oiled baking tray. Bake in the preheated oven for 15 to 20 minutes, until firm and golden. Cool on a wire rack, then store in an airtight container. (Due to the high butter content, try to make these cookies a treat!)

Oatie Cake

Makes 1 cake

15 oz fine oat flour

3 oz raisins

2 tbsp dark brown sugar

2 tsp baking powder

½ tsp ground cinnamon

6 fl oz rice milk

2 organic free-range eggs

pinch of sea salt or to taste

3 oz apple sauce

1 tsp vanilla essence

Preheat the oven to 350°F. Place the dry ingredients in a bowl and mix. Place the wet ingredients in another bowl, whisk together, then stir into the dry ingredients. Turn the mixture into a lightly oiled 9-inch cake pan and bake in the preheated oven for 20 to 30 minutes, until a skewer inserted in the center comes out clean. Turn on to a wire rack and allow to cool before serving.

Mixed Fruit Bread

Makes 1 loaf

6 oz raisins

4 oz golden raisins

2 oz currants

5 oz light or dark brown sugar

½ pint strong cold black tea, strained

1 tbsp soy flour mixed with 1 tbsp filtered water

8 oz plain organic whole-grain flour

1½ tsp baking powder

½ tsp ground allspice

Preheat the oven to 350°F. Place the dried fruit and sugar in a bowl and pour in the tea. Mix well, then soak overnight (or for at least 7 hours). The next day, add the soy flour and water mixture, flour, baking powder and allspice to the fruit and tea mixture. Mix thoroughly with a wooden spoon until all the ingredients are evenly combined. Spoon into a lightly oiled 2-pound loaf tin lined with greaseproof paper and bake in the preheated oven for 1¼ hours or until the teabread has risen and a skewer inserted in the center comes out almost clean. Turn the teabread out of the can and allow it to cool on a wire rack. Wrap it in greaseproof paper and store in an airtight container for 1 to 2 days before eating.

Lemon Walnut Bread

Makes 1 loaf or 24 muffins

3 oz walnuts

12 oz organic whole-grain self-rising flour

2 tsp baking powder

1½ fl oz fresh lemon juice

grated peel of 2 lemons

3 fl oz unsweetened apple juice

3 fl oz sunflower oil

3 fl oz golden syrup or maple syrup

pinch of sea salt or to taste

Preheat the oven to 375°F. Place the walnuts in a heavy bottomed frying pan and toast over a low heat for 5 minutes, stirring frequently. Remove and allow to cool, then chop. Place the lemon juice, lemon peel, apple juice, sunflower oil and golden or maple syrup in a large mixing bowl and beat together. In a separate bowl, mix the flour, baking powder and salt. Now mix the dry ingredients into the wet ingredients, stirring until the batter has become completely smooth. Fold in the walnuts. Pour the batter into a lightly oiled 2-pound loaf pan or partially fill individual paper muffin or cupcake cups in a muffin or cupcake tray. Bake in the preheated oven for 15 minutes, then reduce the heat to 350°F and bake for an additional 20 minutes for a bread loaf, 15 minutes for muffins. Allow to cool before removing the bread from the pan or the muffins from the tray. Serve warm or at room temperature.

Carrot Cake

Makes 1 large or 2 small cakes

1¼ lbs brown rice flour

4 tbsp tapioca, finely ground

1 tbsp ground flaxseeds

8 oz pancake syrup or maple syrup

9 fl oz filtered water

12 oz carrots, grated

6 oz dried figs, finely chopped

1 baking apple, cooked and mashed

1 tbsp baking powder

3 tbsp prune purée

1 tbsp vanilla extract

pinch of sea salt or to taste

Preheat the oven to 350°F. Sift the flour, tapioca and flaxseeds together into a large mixing bowl. Combine the liquids, then stir into the flour mixture. Fold in the remaining ingredients, then pour into a lightly oiled 9x13 inch cake pan or divide between two 10-inch round cans. Bake in the preheated oven for 30 to 40 minutes (longer if using one can). Turn onto a wire rack and allow to cool before serving.

Fig Bars

Makes about 9 bars

> 12 oz dried figs, coarsely chopped
>
> 2 tsp freshly grated lemon zest
>
> 9 fl oz unsweetened apple juice
>
> 3 fl oz sunflower oil
>
> 2 oz fructose or fruit juice sweetener
>
> 6 oz self-rising organic whole-grain flour
>
> 6 oz rolled oats (not instant oatmeal)
>
> 1 tsp baking powder
>
> pinch of sea salt or to taste

Preheat the oven to 350°F. Place the figs, lemon zest and apple juice in a saucepan and bring to a boil. Lower the heat, cover and simmer gently for about 15 minutes, until the figs are tender. Remove from the heat and mash until smooth. Set aside. Place the sunflower oil and fructose or sweetener in a large bowl and mix together. Stir in the remaining ingredients, mixing to a crumb consistency. Press half the crumbly mixture into the bottom of a greaseproof paper-lined cake pan, topping with the fig mixture. Press the remaining crumbly mixture over the filling. Bake in the preheated oven for 40 minutes or until lightly browned. Allow to cool completely before cutting into bars.

Oatie Bran Fingers

Makes 18 fingers

8 oz organic whole-grain flour

3 oz rolled oats

3 oz bran

5 oz dark brown sugar

1 tsp ground ginger

1 tsp ground allspice

3½ oz butter

9 fl oz skim milk

Preheat the oven to 350°F. Place the flour, oats, bran, sugar and spices in a large bowl and mix. Add the butter and rub into the dry ingredients. Stir in the milk to make a stiff dough. Spoon into a greased 6x11-inch cake pan and smooth the surface. Bake in the preheated oven for 25 minutes. Cool in the can, then cut into bars to serve. Store in an airtight container and, due to their high butter content, try not to eat these too often!

SNACKS

French Toast

Serves 4

    1 baking apple, peeled and sliced

    2 tbsp light brown sugar

    3 tbsp flaxseeds

    8 slices whole-grain bread

    3 fl oz filtered water

    6 fl oz unsweetened soy milk

Place the apple slices and sugar in a saucepan and add a little water. Bring to a boil, then simmer gently until the apple is tender. Drain, mash to make apple sauce and set to one side. Grind the flaxseeds in a blender until they turn to powder. Add the water and blend for 1 minute. Beat the flaxseed mixture into the soy milk. Dip the slices of bread in this mixture and cook until browned in a non-stick frying pan. Serve with the apple sauce.

Date Delight

Makes a plateful to share
Submitted by Margaret Gray

    8 oz dates, pitted

    4 oz cottage cheese

Widen the cavity in each date and fill with cottage cheese. Serve as a buffet snack or as a nibble to enjoy while watching TV.

Celery and Cheese

Makes a plateful to share
Submitted by Margaret Gray

    4 celery sticks, washed and chopped into 2-inch lengths
    3 oz cottage cheese
    paprika, as required

Fill the grooves in the celery lengths with cottage cheese and sprinkle paprika over to taste. Serve as a buffet snack or as a TV nibble.

Fruit and Nut Mix

Makes 13 oz

    1 oz dates, chopped
    2 oz raisins, washed
    2 oz unsalted cashews
    2 oz shelled pecans
    2 oz unsalted peanuts
    2 oz sunflower seeds
    2 oz hazelnuts

Mix all the ingredients together and use for snacks. Keep in an airtight container. If stored in the freezer, it will keep for up to 3 months.

BREADS

Wheat Germ Bread

Makes 2 loaves

4 tsp dry yeast

1 tsp sugar

1 pint warm filtered water

1 oz butter

1 lb 6 oz organic whole-grain flour

6 oz wheat germ

1 tsp sea salt

2 tsp malt extract

1 organic free-range egg, beaten

Blend the yeast with the sugar and a little of the warm water and leave for about 20 minutes until frothy. Rub the butter into the flour, wheat germ, salt and malt extract, then make a well in the center. Pour the yeast mixture into it, then stir it in, together with the remaining water, and mix to form a soft dough. Knead well until it is elastic and no longer sticky. Place the dough in an oiled bowl, cover with oiled plastic wrap and leave in a warm place for about an hour, until it has doubled in size. Toward the end of this time, preheat the oven to 450°F. Knead the dough again and divide between two greased 1-pound loaf pans. Leave to rise in a warm place for about 40 minutes, until the dough rises just above the tops of the cans. Brush the tops of the loaves generously with the beaten egg. Bake in the preheated oven for about 30 minutes, until they are golden brown on top and sound hollow when tapped on the base.

Whole-grain Bread

Makes 1 loaf

> 5 oz organic whole-grain flour
> 1 tbsp compressed yeast, loosely crumbled
> 1 tsp sugar
> 2 fl oz lukewarm filtered water
> 1 tsp sea salt
> 1 tsp honey
> 6 fl oz skimmed milk
> sesame or poppy seeds to decorate

Place the yeast, sugar and lukewarm water in a bowl and mix. Stand in a warm place for 5 to 10 minutes until frothy. Mix the flour, salt and honey together in another bowl. Heat the milk gently until it is almost blood temperature, then add the yeast and the milk to flour mixture and stir thoroughly with a wooden spoon until mixed. Knead on a lightly floured surface for 10 minutes or until the dough becomes firm and pliable. Place it in an oiled bowl, covered with oiled plastic wrap, and stand in a warm place for 40 minutes or until the dough has doubled in size. Set the oven to 425°F then knead the dough lightly, mold into the desired shape and stand in a warm place for 10 to 15 minutes. Sprinkle with sesame or poppy seeds. Bake in the oven for 30 minutes.

Banana Bread

Makes 1 cake

> 5 very ripe to overripe bananas
> 2 tbsp dark brown sugar
> 1 tsp vanilla extract
> 12 oz organic whole-grain flour
> 2 tsp baking powder
> ½ tsp bicarbonate of soda
> 2 oz dried fruit (optional)

Preheat the oven to 350°F. Place the bananas, sugar and vanilla in a bowl or blender and mix until smooth. Place the remaining ingredients in another bowl and mix. Add the banana mixture to the dry ingredients and stir well. Spoon into a lightly oiled 8x10-inch cake pan and bake in the preheated oven for about 1 hour or until a skewer inserted in the center comes out almost clean. Turn on to a wire rack and allow to cool.

DRINKS

Fruit Shake

Serves 2–3

> 1 apple, peeled, cored and chopped
> 3 oz cherries, pitted
> 3 oz peaches, peeled, pitted and sliced
> 1 small carton natural live yogurt
> 2 fl oz pineapple, apple or orange juice

Place all the ingredients in a blender, reserving 2 or 3 peach slices or cherries and mix until smooth. Pour into glasses and top with the peach slices or cherries.

Tangy Pink

Serves 2–3

> 1 pink grapefruit, peeled and segmented
> 1 blood orange, peeled and segmented
> 2 tbsp fresh lemon juice

Place the grapefruit and orange segments in a blender and mix. Stir in the lemon juice and pour into glasses.

Green for Go

Serves 2–3

> 1 apple, peeled, cored and quartered
> 5 oz seedless white grapes
> 1 oz fresh coriander, stalks included
> 1 oz watercress
> 1 tbsp fresh lime juice

Place the apple, grapes, coriander and watercress in a blender and mix.
Stir in the lime juice and pour into glasses.

Mint Tea

Makes 10 to 12 glasses

> 4 pints filtered water
> 4 oz mint leaves

Boil the water, then pour it over the leaves in a heatproof bowl. Allow
to stand for 15 minutes. Strain, to remove leaves, then pour the tea into
cups. Drink hot or cold, with ice. Ideally, you should drink all of this
during the course of a couple of days, keeping it in the fridge and
throwing away any left after that time.

Apple Mint

Makes 3 glasses

> 2 peppermint teabags
> 6 fl oz boiling filtered water
> 1 pint apple juice

Place the teabags in the boiling water and allow to stand for 15 minutes. Add the apple juice, allow to cool, then chill in the refrigerator. Serve chilled and drink during the course of a day. For those on the detoxification program only.

Ginger Tea

Makes 4 glasses

> 1½ pints filtered water
> 3-in length fresh ginger root
> two of your favorite tea bags
> fructose to taste

Place the water and ginger root in a saucepan and bring to a boil. Cover and simmer for 5 minutes. Remove from the heat, add the teabags and allow to stand for 5 minutes. Remove the teabags. Strain the ginger from the remaining liquid and add the fructose to taste. Serve warm or chilled, over ice.

Spicy Pineapple Tea

Serves 5

    12 fl oz pineapple juice
    12 fl oz filtered water
    1 tsp whole cloves
    2 cinnamon sticks
    1 lemon, sliced

Place the pineapple juice and water in a saucepan and bring to a boil. Add the cloves, cinnamon and lemon slices and reduce the heat. Cover and simmer for 10 minutes. Remove the cloves and cinnamon before serving hot.

Strawberry Delight

Makes 2–3 glasses

    3 oz strawberries
    6–8 fl oz orange juice
    1 small banana
    1 tsp fructose
    6 ice cubes

Place all the ingredients in a blender and mix until smooth. Serve immediately.

Rice Tea

Serves 2–3

> 2 tbsp brown rice
> 1 pint boiling filtered water
> ½ tsp honey (optional)

Place the rice in a small, heavy bottomed frying pan over a medium heat. Stir the grains until they give out a roasted aroma. Transfer the rice to a small saucepan, add the boiling water and simmer for 1 minute. Cover and turn off the heat. Allow the tea to steep for 3 minutes. Strain and serve hot, with honey, if using.

Fruit Smoothie

Serves 1

> 1 banana, cut into chunks
> 4 oz strawberries
> 2–3 fl oz soy milk or orange juice
> pinch ground cinnamon
> 1–2 ice cubes

Place all the ingredients in a blender and mix until smooth. Serve.

Cran–Apple Tea

Serves 4

> 10 fl oz cranberry juice
>
> 10 fl oz filtered water
>
> 4 herbal teabags (peppermint, cinnamon, lemon and ginger or other flavor of your choice)
>
> 4 cinnamon sticks
>
> 2 tsp honey or to taste

Pour the cranberry juice and water into a medium saucepan and bring to a boil. Add the teabags and cinnamon sticks. Remove from the heat, cover and steep for 5 minutes. Place a cinnamon stick in each of 4 warmed mugs. Pour the tea into the mugs and add honey to taste.

Banarrot Juice

Serves 3–4

> 1 ripe banana, sliced
>
> 2 apples, peeled, cored and chopped
>
> 4 large carrots, chopped
>
> 2 ice cubes (optional)
>
> 2 fl oz apple juice
>
> Place all the ingredients in a blender and mix until smooth. Serve.

Banana Milkshake

Serves 1

> 1 banana, peeled and chopped
>
> 3 oz soft fruit, such as strawberries or raspberries
>
> 4 fl oz carton live natural yogurt
>
> 4–8 tbsp semi-skimmed milk

Place the fruit and yogurt in a blender and mix until smooth. Gradually add the milk until the desired consistency is reached. Serve.

References

Part One

1. R. Dubner and M. A. Ruda (1992) *Trends in Neurological Science* 15, pp. 96–103.

2. Dan Buskila (1997) *Arthritis and Rheumatism Journal*, 40, pp. 446–52.

3. Clifford Woolf (1991) *Pain Journal*, 44, pp. 293–9.

4. H. Moldolfsky (October 1992) Fibromyalgia Association UK, "Fibromyalgia Abstracts."

5. Fibromyalgia Network newsletter (USA) (October 1998).

6. Alan Spanos (January 1998) Fibromyalgia Network newsletter (USA).

7. Fibromyalgia Network newsletter (USA) (October 1998).

8. Knut T. Flytlie and Bjorn F. Madsen (1994) *Q10—Body Fuel*, Forlaget Ny Videnskab (available only from Pharma Nord (UK) Limited, Spital Hall, Mitford, Morpeth NE61 3PN).

9. J. Kleijjnen (November 1992) *Lancet*, vol. 340, no. 8828.

10. D. Warot (1991) "Comparative Effects of Ginkgo Biloba Extracts on Psychomotor Performance and Memory in Healthy Subjects," *Therapie*, no. 46.

Part Two

11. K. J. Pezke, A. Elsner, J. Proll, F. Thielecke and C. C. Metges (2000) *Journal of Nutrition*, 130, pp. 2889–96.

12. A team of Japanese researchers, led by Dr. Yoshiaki Somekawa. See (January 2001) "Obstetrics and Gynecology" newsletter, 97, 1.

13. J. Kleijjnen (November 1992) *Lancet*, 340, 8828.

14. D. Warot (1991) "Comparative Effects of Ginkgo Biloba Extracts on Psychomotor Performance and Memory in Healthy Subjects," *Therapie*, 46.

15. I. J. Russell, J. E. Michalek, J. D. Flechas and G. E. Abraham (1992) "Management of Fibromyalgia: Rationale for the use of Magnesium and Malic Acid," *Journal of Nutritional Medicine*, 3, pp. 49–59.

16. I. J. Russell, J. E. Michalek, J. D. Flechas and G. E. Abraham (1995) "Treatment of FMS with Supermalic: a randomized, double-blind, placebo-controlled crossover pilot study," *Journal of Rheumatology*, 22, pp. 953–8.

Useful Addresses

The American FMS Association
6380 East Tanque Verde
Suite D
Tucson, AZ 85715
Phone: 520-733-1570
Website: www.afsafund.org

The Fibromyalgia Network
PO Box 31750
Tucson, AZ 85751-1750
Phone: 800-853-2929
Fax: 520-290-5550
Website: www.fmnetnews.com
For quarterly newsletters, information and advice.

National Fibromyalgia Association
2200 Glassell Street, Suite '"A"
Orange, CA 92865
Phone: 714-921-0150
Fax: 714-921-6920
Website: www.fmaware.org / e-mail nfa@fmaware.org

Further Reading

Stephen J. Barrett and Ronald E. Gots, *Chemical Sensitivity: The Truth about Environmental Illness*, Prometheus Books, 1998.

Andrew Hall Cutler, *Amalgam Illness, Diagnosis and Treatment: What You Can Do Better, How Your Doctor Can Help You*, Minerva Laboratories, 1999.

Stephen Edelson *Living with Environmental Illness: A Practical Guide to Multiple Chemical Sensitivity*, Taylor Publishing Company, 1998.

Joe Fitzgibbon, *Feeling Tired All the Time*, Gill and Macmillan, London, 2002.

Neil F. Gordon, *Chronic Fatigue: Your Complete Exercise Guide*, Human Kinetics, London, 1993.

Mary Moeller and Karl Moeller, *Fibromyalgia Cookbook*, Fibromyalgia Solutions, 1997.

Barry Sears, *The Zone Diet*, HarperCollins, 1999.

Neville Shone, *Coping Successfully with Pain*, Sheldon Press, London, 1998.

Richard Totman, *Mind, Stress and Health*, Atrium Publishers Group, London, 1991.

Shelley Ann Velekei, *The Fibromyalgia Recipe Book*, Smith Velekei Publishing, 2000.

Index

Other Ulysses Press Mind/Body Titles

ANXIETY & DEPRESSION: A NATURAL APPROACH
2nd edition, Shirley Trickett, $10.95
A step-by-step organic solution for sufferers that puts the reader—not the drugs—in control.

CANDIDA: A NATURAL APPROACH
Shirley Trickett & Karen Brody, $11.95
Shows you how to identify the symptoms and how to avoid habits that encourage candida and other fungal infections.

ENDOMETRIOSIS: A NATURAL APPROACH
Jo Mears, $9.95
Details strategies for managing this distressing disease, including relaxation techniques, meditation, proper diet and pelvic exercises.

FREE YOURSELF FROM TRANQUILIZERS & SLEEPING PILLS: A NATURAL APPROACH
Shirley Trickett, $9.95
Provides a proven step-by-step program for gradual withdrawal from these addictive substances.

IRRITABLE BLADDER & INCONTINENCE: A NATURAL APPROACH
Jennifer Hunt, $8.95
This handy volume offers a simple yet powerful program for taking control of your life.

MIGRAINES: A NATURAL APPROACH
2nd edition, Sue Dyson, $12.95
Offers easy-to-understand explanations and holistic treatments to this major health problem.

PANIC ATTACKS: A NATURAL APPROACH
2nd edition, Shirley Trickett, $9.95
Demystifies this condition and shows how to stop pressing the panic button.

50+ YOGA: TIPS AND TECHNIQUES FOR A SAFE AND HEALTHY PRACTICE
Richard Rosen, $12.95

Focusing on the needs of the beginning student 50 years and older, this book details the basic principles of yoga and teaches the yoga poses through the use of step-by-step photos, clearly written instructions and helpful hints.

HOW MEDITATION HEALS: A SCIENTIFIC EXPLANATION
Eric Harrison, $12.95

In straightforward, practical terms, *How Meditation Heals* reveals how and why meditation improves the natural functioning of the human body.

KNOW YOUR BODY: THE ATLAS OF ANATOMY
2nd edition, Introduction by Emmet B. Keeffe, M.D., $14.95

Provides a comprehensive, full-color guide to the human body.

PILATES WORKBOOK: ILLUSTRATED STEP-BY-STEP GUIDE
TO MATWORK TECHNIQUES
Michael King, $12.95

Illustrates the core matwork movements exactly as Joseph Pilates intended them to be performed; readers learn each movement by simply following the photographic sequences and explanatory captions.

YOGA THERAPIES: 45 SEQUENCES TO RELIEVE STRESS, DEPRESSION,
REPETITIVE STRAIN, SPORTS INJURIES AND MORE
Jessie Chapman   Photographs by Dhyan, $14.95

Featuring an inspiring artistic presentation, this book is filled with beautifully photographed sequences that relieve stress, release anger, relax back muscles and reverse repetitive strain injuries.

To order these books call 800-377-2542 or 510-601-8301, fax 510-601-8307, e-mail ulysses@ulyssespress.com, or write to Ulysses Press, P.O. Box 3440, Berkeley, CA 94703. All retail orders are shipped free of charge. California residents must include sales tax. Allow two to three weeks for delivery.

About the Author

Christine Craggs-Hinton, mother of three strapping sons, followed a career in the Civil Service until severe post-traumatic pain forced her into early retirement. Since being diagnosed as having fibromyalgia in 1992, she has directed her remaining energies into researching the condition. In 1997, she became a committee member of the newly established Fibromyalgia Support and Carers' Group (West Yorkshire), and for a year edited their newsletters. In 1999, she began contributing to the Fibromyalgia Association UK newsletters, and now writes regularly for the monthly ukfibromyalgia.com *FaMily* magazine.